Transforming Eight Deadly Emotions into Healthy Ones

C   >rked in psy-
c   or editor of
ovei   999), *Self-discipline: How to get it and how to keep it* (Sheldon Press, 2009), *Coping with Life's Challenges: Moving on from adversity* (Sheldon Press, 2010), *Coping with Envy* (Sheldon Press, 2010), *How to Develop Inner Strength* (Sheldon Press, 2011) and *Coping with Manipulation* (Sheldon Press, 2011).

Overcoming Common Problems Series

Selected titles

A full list of titles is available from Sheldon Press,
36 Causton Street, London SW1P 4ST and on our website at
www.sheldonpress.co.uk

101 Questions to Ask Your Doctor
Dr Tom Smith

Birth Over 35
Sheila Kitzinger

Bulimia, Binge-eating and their Treatment
Professor J. Hubert Lacey, Dr Bryony Bamford
and Amy Brown

Coeliac Disease: What you need to know
Alex Gazzola

Coping Successfully with Shyness
Margaret Oakes, Professor Robert Bor
and Dr Carina Eriksen

Coping with Anaemia
Dr Tom Smith

Coping with Asthma in Adults
Mark Greener

Coping wth Bronchitis and Emphysema
Dr Tom Smith

Coping with Drug Problems in the Family
Lucy Jolin

Coping with Dyspraxia
Jill Eckersley

Coping with Early-onset Dementia
Jill Eckersley

Coping with Envy
Dr Windy Dryden

Coping with Gout
Christine Craggs-Hinton

**Coping with Manipulation: When others
blame you for their feelings**
Dr Windy Dryden

**Coping with Obsessive Compulsive
Disorder**
Professor Kevin Gournay, Rachel Piper
and Professor Paul Rogers

Coping with Stomach Ulcers
Dr Tom Smith

Depressive Illness: The curse of the strong
Dr Tim Cantopher

**Divorce and Separation: A legal guide
for all couples**
Dr Mary Welstead

Dying for a Drink
Dr Tim Cantopher

**Epilepsy: Complementary and alternative
treatements**
Dr Sallie Baxendale

The Heart Attack Survival Guide
Mark Greener

High-risk Body Size: Take control of your weight
Dr Funké Barrour

How to Beat Worry and Stress
Dr David Devlin

How to Develop Inner Strength
Dr Windy Dryden

**Let's Stay Together: A guide to lasting
relationships**
Jane Butterworth

Living with IBS
Nuno Ferreira and David T. Gillanders

**Living with a Problem Drinker:
Your survival guide**
Rolande Anderson

Living with Tinnitus and Hyperacusis
Dr Laurence McKenna, Dr David Baguley
and Dr Don McFerran

Losing a Parent
Fiona Marshall

Making Sense of Trauma: How to tell your story
Dr Nigel C. Hunt and Dr Sue McHale

Motor Neurone Disease: A family affair
Dr David Oliver

Natural Treatment for Arthritis
Christine Craggs-Hinton

**Overcoming Gambling: A guide for problem
and compulsive gamblers**
Philip Mawer

Overcoming Loneliness
Alice Muir

**The Pain Management Handbook:
Your personal guide**
Neville Shone

Reducing Your Risk of Dementia
Dr Tom Smith

**Therapy for Beginners: How to get the best
out of counselling**
Professor Robert Bor, Sheila Gill and Anne Stokes

**Transforming Eight Deadly Emotions
into Healthy Ones**
Dr Windy Dryden

Treating Arthritis: The drug-free way
Margaret Hills and Christine Horner

Treating Arthritis: The supplements guide
Julia Davies

Overcoming Common Problems

Transforming Eight Deadly Emotions into Healthy Ones

DR WINDY DRYDEN

sheldon PRESS

First published in Great Britain in 2012

Sheldon Press
36 Causton Street
London SW1P 4ST
www.sheldonpress.co.uk

British Library Cataloguing-in-Publication Data
A catalogue record for this book is available from the British Library

ISBN 978-1-84709-134-5
eBook ISBN 978-1-84709-248-9

Typeset by Caroline Waldron, Wirral, Cheshire
Printed in Great Britain by Ashford Colour Press
Subsequently digitally printed in Great Britain

Produced on paper from sustainable forests

Contents

You know, sometimes we're not prepared for adversity
When it happens, sometimes we're caught short
We don't know exactly how to handle it when it comes up
Sometimes, we don't know . . . just what to do when adversity takes over
I have advice for all of us. I got it from my pianist, Joe Zawinul,
who wrote this tune
And it sounds like what you're supposed to say when you have
that kind of problem
It's called: Mercy, Mercy, Mercy . . .

(Cannonball Adderley's verbal introduction to 'Mercy, Mercy, Mercy', 1966)

Preface

In this book, I am going to consider the eight emotional problems that people routinely seek help for and how you can deal with them. I wanted to discuss all eight problems in one volume, since many of you will experience more than one such emotional problem during your lives. I call these emotional problems 'deadly' emotions not because they will kill you, but because they probably have a detrimental effect on your well-being.

I begin the book by outlining the foundations of emotional problems. I then devote one chapter to each of the eight deadly emotions and use a similar structure in each chapter. Thus, I will start by helping you to understand the deadly emotion in question, discuss what you disturb yourself about when you experience it, and outline what largely determines the emotion and how you tend to act and think when you experience it. Next, I will discuss how you can deal with the deadly emotion in question. I will help you to identify the themes in the emotion, and your behaviour and thinking when you experience it, before encouraging you to set appropriate emotional, behavioural and thinking goals. Then, I will help you to identify, challenge and change the rigid and extreme beliefs that account for your emotional problem and to develop the flexible and non-extreme beliefs that will enable you to achieve your goals. After this, I will show you what you need to do to strengthen your conviction in your rational beliefs so that you become less prone to your deadly emotion. I will then deal with a number of additional issues relevant to the deadly emotion in question before finally outlining a number of world views that underpin the deadly emotion and its healthy alternative.

The common chapter structure that I employ in Chapters 2–9 is to ensure that all relevant issues are discussed for each deadly emotion. As I said at the outset, while it is unlikely that you will be prone to all eight deadly emotions you may be prone to two or three. The view of emotional problems that I am taking in this book states that while there are common features among the eight deadly emotions, there are also features that are distinctive to each emotion. This is reflected in Chapters 2–9 and you will need to bear this point in mind when you read these chapters or a selection of them.

Windy Dryden
London and Eastbourne

1
The deadly emotions: an introduction

In this book, I'm going to discuss some common emotional problems (or what I refer to here as 'deadly emotions') and show you how to deal with them. In my previous emotion-focused books for Sheldon Press, I devoted one book to each of the eight deadly emotions for which people routinely seek help. However, as many people experience more than one deadly emotion, I decided to write a popular self-help book that covers all eight deadly emotions so you can focus on the emotions you are particularly plagued by.

In this opening chapter, I'm going to cover some very important material that I regard as foundations to your understanding of the deadly emotions and the healthy alternatives to them.

What are the eight deadly emotions?

The eight deadly emotions that I will cover in this book are:

- anxiety
- depression
- guilt
- shame
- hurt
- unhealthy anger
- unhealthy jealousy
- unhealthy envy.

What are healthy alternatives to the eight deadly emotions?

When you experience a deadly emotion it is in response to a negative life event or adversity. Adversity[1] is unfortunately a fact of life, so when you're looking for a healthy alternative to a deadly emotion in the face

---

1 Throughout this book, I will refer to events where you don't get what you want or get what you don't want as 'adversities'.

of adversity, it isn't realistic for that emotion to be positive or neutral. It is realistic for that emotion to be negative, but healthy.

Healthy negative emotions as healthy alternatives to the deadly emotions

Healthy alternatives to deadly emotions are known as 'healthy negative emotions'. This term is used for two good reasons. First, such emotions have a negative tone and this is their realistic aspect. Remember that we're talking about emotions in the context of life's adversities. It is realistic to feel a negative emotion about a negative event. Second, such emotions are healthy in that they are associated with a different set of behaviours and ways of thinking than are the deadly emotions. I will discuss this in greater detail later in this chapter. For now, here is the list of healthy negative emotions:[2]

- concern (rather than anxiety)
- sadness (rather than depression)
- remorse (rather than guilt)
- disappointment (rather than shame)
- sorrow (rather than hurt)
- healthy anger (rather than unhealthy anger)
- healthy jealousy (rather than unhealthy jealousy)
- healthy envy (rather than unhealthy envy).

Rational-Emotive Cognitive Behavioural Therapy

This book is based on Rational-Emotive Cognitive Behavioural Therapy. You may have heard of Cognitive Behaviour Therapy (CBT) and it being described as a therapeutic approach. However, in my view, CBT is not a therapeutic approach but a therapeutic tradition in which there are a number of distinct approaches, of which Rational-Emotive Behaviour Therapy (known as REBT) is one. REBT was founded in 1955 by Dr Albert Ellis (1913–2007). The term 'Rational-Emotive Cognitive Behaviour Therapy' (RECBT) – which I'll use in this book to remind you of the book's legacy – shows that RECBT is placed within the CBT tradition and that its distinctive features are rooted in REBT.

The eight deadly emotions are underpinned by irrational beliefs

RECBT theory argues that each of the eight deadly emotions stems from two irrational beliefs (IBs): a rigid belief and a group of three extreme

---

2 We do not have agreed terms for healthy negative emotions. Thus, it is important that you use the terms that are meaningful to you rather than the terms in this list.

beliefs derived from the rigid belief. Thus, an IB is characterized by being rigid or being extreme. It has three other characteristics: (1) it is false; (2) it is illogical; and (3) it has largely unconstructive consequences (e.g. in the face of an adversity it leads to a deadly emotion).

Let me consider rigid and extreme beliefs separately.

Rigid beliefs

Perhaps the most basic characteristic of human beings is that we have desires. We want certain things to happen and other things not to happen, but when we turn these desires into rigidities and we don't get what we want or get what we don't want, then we experience one or more of the deadly emotions described in this book. Here are a few examples of rigid beliefs:

- I must do well on the forthcoming test.
- You must respect my boundaries.
- The world must not give me too much hassle.

As these examples show, you can hold rigid beliefs about yourself, others and life conditions.

Three extreme beliefs

According to RECBT theory, rigid beliefs are paramount in explaining the existence of the deadly emotions and three extreme beliefs tend to be derived from these rigid beliefs. These are (1) awfulizing beliefs; (2) discomfort intolerance beliefs; and (3) depreciation beliefs.

Awfulizing beliefs   An awfulizing belief stems from the rigid belief that things mustn't be as bad as they are. An awfulizing belief is extreme in the sense that you believe *at the time* one or more of the following:

1 Nothing could be worse.
2 The event in question is worse than 100 per cent bad.
3 No good could possibly come from this bad event.

In the following examples of awfulizing beliefs, the rigid beliefs are listed in brackets.

- (I must do well on the forthcoming test) . . . and it will be awful if I don't.
- (You must respect my boundaries) . . . and it's the end of the world when you don't.
- (The world must not give me too much hassle) . . . and it's terrible when it does.

Discomfort intolerance beliefs   A discomfort intolerance belief stems from a rigid belief that things must not be as frustrating or uncomfortable as they are. A discomfort intolerance belief is extreme in the sense that you believe *at the time* one or more of the following:

1 I will die or disintegrate if the frustration or discomfort continues to exist.
2 I will lose the capacity to experience happiness if the frustration or discomfort continues to exist.

In the following examples of discomfort intolerance beliefs, the rigid beliefs are listed in brackets.

- (I must do well on the forthcoming test) . . . and I won't be able to bear it if I don't.
- (You must respect my boundaries) . . . and it's intolerable if you don't.
- (The world must not give me too much hassle) . . . and I can't stand it if it does.

Depreciation beliefs   A depreciation belief stems from the rigid belief that you, others or things must be as you want them to be and is extreme in the sense that you believe *at the time* one or more of the following:

1 A person (self or other) can legitimately be given a single global rating that defines his or her essence and the worth of a person is dependent upon conditions that change (e.g. my worth goes up when I do well and goes down when I don't do well).
2 The world can legitimately be given a single rating that defines its essential nature, and the value of the world varies according to what happens within it (e.g. the value of the world goes up when something fair occurs and goes down when something unfair happens).
3 A person can be rated on the basis of one of his or her aspects and the world can be rated on the basis of one of its aspects.

In the following examples of depreciation beliefs, the rigid beliefs are listed in brackets.

- (I must do well on the forthcoming test) . . . and I'm a failure if I don't.
- (You must respect my boundaries) . . . and you're bad if you don't.
- (The world must not give me too much hassle) . . . and if it does, the world is a rotten place.

The healthy alternatives to the eight deadly emotions are underpinned by rational beliefs

RECBT theory argues that each of the eight healthy alternatives to the deadly emotions stems from two rational beliefs (RBs): a flexible belief and a group of three non-extreme beliefs that are derived from the flexible belief. Thus, an RB is characterized by being flexible or being non-extreme. It has three other characteristics: (1) it is true; (2) it is logical; and (3) it has largely constructive consequences (e.g. in the face of an adversity it leads to a healthy negative emotion).

Let me consider flexible and non-extreme beliefs separately.

Flexible beliefs

As I pointed out earlier in this chapter, it is a basic characteristic of human beings that we have desires. We want certain things to happen and other things not to happen. When we keep these desires flexible and we don't get what we want or get what we don't want, then we experience one or more of the healthy negative emotions outlined earlier. Here are a few examples of flexible beliefs:

- I would like to do well on the forthcoming test, but I don't have to do so.
- I want you to respect my boundaries, but unfortunately you don't have to do so.
- I would prefer it if the world did not give me too much hassle, but the world does not have to be the way I want it to be.

As these examples show, you can hold flexible beliefs about yourself, others and life conditions. You will note from these examples that flexible beliefs have two components: (1) an 'asserted preference' component (e.g. 'I would like to do well on the forthcoming test . . .') and (2) a 'negated rigid' component (e.g. '. . . but I don't have to do so').

Three non-extreme beliefs

According to RECBT theory, flexible beliefs are paramount in explaining the existence of healthy negative emotions and three non-extreme beliefs tend to be derived from these flexible beliefs. These are (1) non-awfulizing beliefs; (2) discomfort tolerance beliefs; and (3) acceptance beliefs.

Non-awfulizing beliefs   A non-awfulizing belief stems from the flexible belief that you would like things not to be as bad as they are, but that doesn't mean that they must not be as bad. This belief is non-extreme in the sense that you believe *at the time* one or more of the following:

1 Things could always be worse.
2 The event in question is less than 100 per cent bad.
3 Good could come from this bad event.

In the following examples of non-awfulizing beliefs, the flexible beliefs are listed in brackets.

• (I would like to do well on the forthcoming test, but I don't have to do so) . . . and if I don't do well, it will be bad, but not awful.
• (I want you to respect my boundaries, but unfortunately you don't have to do so) . . . It's disadvantageous to me if you don't, but not the end of the world.
• (I would prefer it if the world did not give me too much hassle, but the world doesn't have to be the way I want it to be) . . . It's bad when it's not, but not terrible.

You will note from these examples that non-awfulizing beliefs have two components: (1) an 'asserted badness' component (e.g. 'If I don't do well on the forthcoming test, it will be bad . . .') and a 'negated awfulizing' component (e.g. '. . . but it wouldn't be awful').

Discomfort tolerance beliefs A discomfort tolerance belief stems from the flexible belief that it is undesirable when things are as frustrating or uncomfortable as they are, but unfortunately things don't have to be different. A discomfort tolerance belief is non-extreme in the sense that you believe *at the time* one or more of the following:

1 I will struggle if the frustration or discomfort continues to exist, but I will neither die nor disintegrate.
2 I will not lose the capacity to experience happiness if the frustration or discomfort continues to exist, although this capacity will be temporarily diminished.
3 The frustration or discomfort is worth tolerating.

In the following examples of discomfort tolerance beliefs, the flexible beliefs are listed in brackets.

• (I would like to do well on the forthcoming test, but I don't have to do so) . . . It will be a struggle for me if I don't do well, but I could bear it and it would be worth bearing.
• (I want you to respect my boundaries, but unfortunately you don't have to do so) . . . It's hard for me to bear it if you don't respect my boundaries, but I can tolerate it and it is in my interests to do so.
• (I would prefer it if the world did not give me too much hassle, but the world doesn't have to be the way I want it to be) . . . When it is not the way I want, it is difficult for me to tolerate it, but I can stand it and it's worthwhile for me to do so.

You will note from these examples that discomfort tolerance beliefs have three components: (1) an 'asserted struggle' component (e.g. 'It will be a struggle for me if I don't do well on the forthcoming test . . .'); (2) a 'negated unbearability' component (e.g. '. . . but I could bear it . . .'); and (3) a 'worth it' component (e.g. '. . . and it would be worth bearing').

Acceptance beliefs An acceptance belief stems from a flexible belief that it is preferable but not necessary that you, others or things are the way you want them to be, and is non-extreme in the sense that you believe *at the time* one or more of the following:

1 A person cannot legitimately be given a single global rating that defines his or her essence, and that person's worth, as far as he or she has it, is not dependent upon conditions that change (e.g. 'My worth stays the same whether or not I do well').
2 The world cannot legitimately be given a single rating that defines its essential nature, and the value of the world does not vary according to what happens within it (e.g. the value of the world stays the same whether fairness exists at any given time or not).
3 It makes sense to rate discrete aspects of a person and of the world, but it does not make sense to rate a person or the world on the basis of these discrete aspects.

In the following examples of acceptance beliefs, the flexible beliefs are listed in brackets.

- (I would like to do well on the forthcoming test, but I don't have to do so) . . . If I don't do well, it's bad, but I am not a failure. I am an unrateable, fallible human being capable of doing well and poorly on tests.
- (I want you to respect my boundaries, but unfortunately you don't have to do so) . . . If you don't, you are not a bad person; rather, you are an ordinary human being capable of doing good, bad and neutral things.
- (I would prefer it if the world did not give me too much hassle, but the world does not have to be the way I want it to be) . . . When the world does give me more hassle than I want, it isn't a rotten place; rather, it is a complex mixture of good, bad and neutral aspects.

You will note from these examples that acceptance beliefs have three components: (1) an 'aspect evaluation' component (e.g. 'If I don't do well, it's bad . . .'); (2) a 'negated depreciation' component (e.g. '. . . but I'm not a failure'; and (3) an 'asserted acceptance' component (e.g. '. . . I am an unrateable, fallible human being capable of doing well and poorly on tests').

Inference themes in relation to your personal domain

While deadly emotions and healthy negative emotions can be differentiated in general by the beliefs that underpin them (irrational in the first case, rational in the second), in order to distinguish between particular deadly emotions and their specific healthy alternatives we need to understand a concept known as inference themes, as these relate to an individual's personal domain. Let me discuss the concept of personal domain first.

Personal domain

The concept known as the personal domain first appeared in the psychological literature in 1976 in an excellent book entitled *Cognitive Therapy and the Emotional Disorders* by Dr A.T. Beck, one of the grandfathers of Cognitive Behaviour Therapy (CBT). Your personal domain has three features:

- Your personal domain contains people, objects and ideas in which you have an involvement.
- Your personal domain is like an onion in that these people, objects and ideas can occupy a central, intermediate and peripheral place within it.
- There are two basic areas within your personal domain – an ego area and a comfort area. As you will see, six of the eight deadly emotions that I discuss in this book can be related to one or both areas, while two of them (i.e. shame and guilt) appear to be related only to the ego area.

Inference

An inference is an interpretation that you make about a situation that goes beyond the data at hand that has personal meaning to you. An inference may be accurate or inaccurate and needs to be tested against the available evidence. Often you do not know for certain whether an inference that you have made is accurate or inaccurate, and therefore the best you can do is to make the 'best bet' given the data at hand. The accuracy of an inference often becomes clear after you have made it. This is particularly the case when you make an inference about a future event.

Inference theme

As you will see from the forthcoming chapters, when you experience one of the following pairs of emotions, each emotion pairing is related to a specific theme or themes related to your personal domain: anxiety vs concern; depression vs sadness; shame vs disappointment; guilt vs remorse; hurt vs sorrow; unhealthy anger vs healthy anger; unhealthy jealousy vs healthy jealousy; and unhealthy envy vs healthy envy. I will discuss and illustrate the specific themes in the relevant chapters.

Distinguishing deadly emotions from their healthy alternatives

In this section, I will discuss in general how you can reliably distinguish deadly emotions from their healthy alternatives. In each of the chapters that follow I will discuss in detail how to distinguish the deadly emotion in question, with its specific healthy alternative.

Inference themes and beliefs

We know from the above that inference themes show you which of the eight emotional pairings you are experiencing (e.g. when your inference theme is threat, you experience either anxiety or concern), but on their own they do not help you to distinguish which emotion you are experiencing within the pairing (i.e. you cannot tell by the inference theme of threat alone whether your emotion is anxiety or concern).

We also know that when you hold an IB about an adversity (but we do not know the inference theme of that adversity) then your emotion will be deadly, but we don't know which of the eight deadly emotions you are experiencing. Conversely, we know that when you hold an RB about an adversity (again, we do not know the inference theme of that adversity) then your emotion will be a healthy negative one, but again we don't know which of the eight healthy negative emotions you are experiencing.

However, when we combine these two pieces of information then we are in a better position to distinguish specific deadly emotions from their healthy alternatives. For example, if we know that the theme of your adversity is threat and you hold an IB about that threat, then we are well placed to conclude that you are experiencing anxiety. Similarly, if we know that the theme of your adversity is threat and you hold an RB about that threat, then we are well placed to conclude that you are experiencing concern. Putting this more succinctly:

Inference theme	Rationality of belief	Emotion
Threat	Irrational	Anxiety
Threat	Rational	Concern

Associated behaviour

So far, I have mentioned that one way of distinguishing between a deadly emotion and its healthy negative emotion alternative is to take the theme of what the person has feelings about with respect to the adversity that he or she is facing and the belief that the person holds that accounts for the emotion. You have learned the following:

Adversity inference theme + Irrational belief = Deadly emotion

Adversity inference theme + Rational belief = Healthy negative emotion

Now, when you hold a belief about an adversity you don't just experience an emotion, you also experience a tendency to act in a certain way (known as an action tendency) which you may or may not convert into overt behaviour.

Thus, another way to tell if what you feel in a specific situation is a deadly emotion or a healthy negative emotion is to examine how you acted or, if you did not take action, to examine your action tendency.

Barbara was angry with her boss when he did not recommend her for promotion, an advancement which she believed she thoroughly deserved. Barbara considered that her boss had acted in a very unfair manner towards her. She was unsure whether her anger was negative and unhealthy or negative but healthy, so she considered how she acted in the situation. This did not help her because she did not take any action when she discovered the news, or subsequently. Finally, she considered what she felt like doing but did not do. Barbara's action tendency was to scream abuse at her boss and to get revenge against him by getting him into trouble with his boss. Such action tendencies were clearly hostile in nature and showed Barbara that her anger was an emotional problem.

Associated thinking

The final way of determining whether you are experiencing a deadly emotion or a healthy negative emotion about an adversity is to inspect the thinking that is associated with the emotion. This is different from the inference that you made about the situation that constituted your adversity. Such thinking has not yet been processed by your beliefs. The thinking that I am referring to here is the thinking that is associated with your emotion. This is the thinking that has been produced when your adversity has been processed by your beliefs. When your adversity has been processed by IBs then the thinking that results is very likely to be highly distorted and skewed to the negative in content and ruminative in nature. However, when this adversity has been processed by RBs then the thinking that results is very likely to be realistic and balanced in content and non-ruminative in nature. David Burns, a leading cognitive therapist, in his book *Feeling Good: The new mood therapy* (William Morrow, 1980) first outlined a list of thinking errors – which are by nature highly distorted and skewed to the negative – that people make when they have processed adversities with IBs. I outline and illustrate some of these thinking errors and their realistic and balanced alternatives in

Appendix 1. You should consult this list if you are unsure whether the thinking you engage in when you are experiencing an emotion is realistic and balanced or highly distorted and skewed to the negative.

Helen (a co-worker of Barbara's) was also angry with her boss when he did not recommend her for promotion, an advancement which she believed she thoroughly deserved. Helen considered that her boss had acted in a very unfair manner towards her. Helen was unsure whether her anger was deadly or negative but healthy, so she considered how she thought in the situation. She thought about asserting herself with her boss after planning what to say. After she had done this she made an appointment to see her boss and, in the days that followed until the meeting, she thought about the issue in passing, but did not ruminate on it. Given that Helen's thinking that went along with her anger was realistic and balanced and non-ruminative, she considered that her anger was a healthy negative emotion and not a deadly emotion.

Let me take the points that I have made in this section and the previous one on behaviour and add it to the material that I presented on p. 10.

Adversity inference theme + Irrational belief	= Deadly emotion Unconstructive behaviour and action tendencies Highly distorted thinking that is skewed to the negative and ruminative in nature
Adversity inference theme + Rational belief	= Healthy negative emotion Constructive behaviour and action tendencies Realistic and balanced thinking that is non-ruminative in nature

In the chapters that follow, I will employ a similar structure. First, I will outline the major factors that need to be considered when understanding the deadly emotion under focus. Second, I will show you what steps you need to take in order to change each deadly emotion to its healthy negative emotion. Finally, I will discuss what you need to do to make yourself less prone to whatever deadly emotions you are particularly susceptible to. I will begin by considering one of the most common deadly emotions, anxiety.

2

Dealing with anxiety

Anxiety is perhaps the most prevalent emotional problem and certainly one of the two most common problems for which people seek help (depression being the other). In this chapter, I outline the RECBT view of anxiety and its healthy alternative, concern, before showing you how to deal effectively with this deadly emotion.

Understanding anxiety

In this section, I discuss the RECBT view of what happens when you make yourself anxious and how to deal effectively with this deadly emotion. In doing so I will use RECBT's 'ABC' model where 'A' stands for 'adversity', 'B' for beliefs and 'C' for the consequences of these beliefs. However, I will use the order 'CAB' since it's best to start with features of anxiety at 'C'.

'C'

Chapter 1 showed the three main features of any emotional problem: feeling, behavioural and thinking. When anxious, you are likely feel this emotion in several ways. Common experiences include rapid breathing, increased heart rate, trembling, nausea, going red, a general feeling of not being in control. These feelings may interfere with your thinking clearly about the threat you face or think you face, and impede constructive action.

Behaviour associated with anxiety

When anxious, you are motivated to take steps designed to keep you safe. Table 2.1 outlines the major ways you act or feel like acting when anxious.

Thinking associated with anxiety

When anxious, you may think in one of two ways:

- engaging in thinking designed to keep you safe; or
- exaggerating in your mind the threat you face (or think you face) and its consequences (see Table 2.1).

You can rapidly switch from one type of thinking to the other.

Table 2.1 Anxiety vs concern

Adversity	• You are facing a threat to your personal domain.	
Belief	IRRATIONAL	RATIONAL
Emotion	Anxiety	Concern
Behaviour	• You avoid the threat. • You withdraw physically from the threat. • You ward off the threat (e.g. by rituals or superstitious behaviour). • You try to neutralize the threat (e.g. by being nice to people of whom you are afraid). • You distract yourself from the threat by engaging in other activity. • You keep checking on the current status of the threat, hoping to find that it has disappeared or become benign. • You seek reassurance from others that the threat is benign. • You seek support from others so that if the threat happens they will handle it or be there to rescue you. • You over-prepare in order to minimize the threat happening or so that you are prepared to meet it (NB: it is the over-preparation that is the problem here). • You tranquillize your feelings so that you don't think about the threat. • You overcompensate for feeling vulnerable by seeking out an even greater threat to prove to yourself that you can cope.	• You face up to the threat without using any safety-seeking measures. • You take constructive action to deal with the threat. • You seek support from others to help you face up to the threat and then take constructive action by yourself rather than relying on them to handle it for you or to be there to rescue you. • You prepare to meet the threat but do not over-prepare.
Subsequent thinking	*Threat-exaggerating thinking* • You overestimate the probability of the threat occurring. • You underestimate your	• You are realistic about the probability of the threat occurring. • You view the threat realistically.

ability to cope with the threat.
- You ruminate about the threat.
- You create an even more negative threat in your mind.
- You magnify the negative consequences of the threat and minimize its positive consequences.
- You have more task-irrelevant thoughts than in concern.

Safety-seeking thinking
- You withdraw mentally from the threat.
- You try to persuade yourself that the threat is not imminent and that you are 'imagining' it.
- You think in ways designed to reassure yourself that the threat is benign or, if not, that its consequences will be insignificant.
- You distract yourself from the threat, e.g. by focusing on mental scenes of safety and well-being.
- You over-prepare mentally in order to minimize the threat happening or so that you are prepared to meet it (NB: once again it is the over-preparation that is the problem here).
- You picture yourself dealing with the threat in a masterful way.
- You overcompensate for your feeling of vulnerability by picturing yourself dealing effectively with an even bigger threat.

- You realistically appraise your ability to cope with the threat.
- You think about what to do concerning dealing with the threat constructively rather than ruminate about the threat.
- You have more task-relevant thoughts than in anxiety.

'A'

Recall from Chapter 1 that 'A' stands for adversity – what you are most disturbed about with respect to your personal domain. When anxious, you face (or think you face) some kind of threat to a key aspect of your personal domain. A threat relates to something that hasn't happened yet but is imminent in actuality or when you think about it.

Threats to the ego realm of your personal domain

When you experience 'ego anxiety', the threat you face (or think you face) concerns the ego realm of your personal domain (or your self-esteem). Examples of ego threats include the prospect of:

- being criticized
- being negatively evaluated by others
- being rejected
- being disapproved of
- being rejected
- failing
- losing your job.

Threats to the non-ego realm of the personal domain

When you experience 'non-ego anxiety', the threat you face (or think you face) concerns the non-ego realm of your personal domain (your sense of comfort, broadly defined). Examples of non-ego threats include:

- being uncertain you are not safe from threat

and the prospect of:

- beginning to lose self-control;
- experiencing discomfort due to interpersonal conflict;
- experiencing uncomfortable emotions;
- being frustrated in pursuit of an important goal;
- losing your job.

Notice that the prospect of losing your job is listed as both an ego threat and a non-ego threat, showing that the same adversity may pose a threat to both ego and non-ego realms of your personal domain.

'B'

As Chapter 1 explained, beliefs are at the heart of the RECBT model of the emotions. Thus threats to your personal domain on their own don't explain your anxiety, since, as you'll see, it's possible and desirable for you to feel concerned about these threats. Chapter 1 showed how you can hold a set of irrational beliefs (IBs) or rational beliefs (RBs) about threat.

Irrational beliefs about threat

The RECBT model of anxiety is that you feel anxious about threats to your personal domain when you hold IBs about threat. These beliefs are rigid and extreme. Please note:

- rigid beliefs are common to both ego anxiety and non-ego anxiety;
- self-depreciation beliefs are the main extreme beliefs in ego anxiety;
- awfulizing beliefs or discomfort intolerance beliefs are the main extreme beliefs in non-ego anxiety.

Understanding concern

As Chapter 1 explained, when you face a negative event it is healthy to experience a negative emotion that helps you deal effectively with the negative event you face. In this section I discuss the RECBT view of concern as the healthy alternative to anxiety. Again I use the 'CABDE' order of the 'ABCDE' framework (where D = disputing irrational beliefs and E = effects of disputing).

'C'

As mentioned above, there are three main features of anxiety: feeling, behavioural and thinking. The same is true when you're concerned but not anxious. When concerned, you may have butterflies in your tummy and your breathing may be increased, but not as much as when you're anxious. These feelings encourage you to think clearly about the threat and motivate you to take constructive action.

Behaviour associated with concern

When concerned but not anxious, you are motivated to face the threat and deal with it. Table 2.1 outlines the major ways you act or feel like acting when you are concerned.

Thinking associated with concern

When concerned but not anxious, you tend to think in ways designed to help you face and deal effectively with the threat (see Table 2.1).

'A'

When you are concerned about the threats about which you previously felt anxious, these threats are the same (see Table 2.1).

'B'

When you feel concerned but not anxious about a threat, you do so because the beliefs you hold about the threat are rational.

Rational beliefs about threat

The RECBT model of concern is that you feel concerned but not anxious about threats to your personal domain when you hold RBs about threat. These beliefs are flexible and non-extreme. Please note:

- flexible beliefs are common to both ego concern and non-ego concern;
- unconditional self-acceptance beliefs are the main non-extreme beliefs in ego concern;
- non-awfulizing beliefs or discomfort tolerance beliefs are the main non-extreme beliefs in non-ego concern.

How to deal with anxiety

Since you make yourself anxious about a particular threat, your goal is to make yourself concerned but not anxious about the same threat. That's why I'll be encouraging you to assume temporarily that your inferences of threat at 'A' are correct. Once you are concerned rather than anxious, you will be in a sufficiently rational frame of mind to examine your threat-related inferences. If you're anxious about threat you will not be objective enough while examining your inferences. I will explain later why you are prone to inferring the existence of threat in ambiguous situations and will help you become less prone.

Ensure that you are feeling anxious and it's a problem for you

Before you do anything to try to change your feelings of anxiety, ensure that you are anxious; if so, you should see that anxiety is a problem for you. Otherwise, you will resist your own efforts to help yourself.

Are you anxious?

People use the term 'anxiety' quite loosely, and if you say you're anxious you may or may not be experiencing the deadly version of this emotion. One good way of determining whether or not you are experiencing the deadly version is by consulting the behavioural and thinking consequences of both IBs and RBs about threat (see Table 2.1). The more your behaviour and thinking match those listed in that table as consequences of IBs, the more likely you are/were anxious rather than concerned. Conversely, the more your behaviour and thinking match those listed as consequences of RBs, the more likely you are/were concerned rather than anxious.

Is your anxiety a problem for you?

Assuming you have determined that you experienced anxiety rather than concern, the next step is to determine whether or not you consider your anxiety a problem for you which you want to change. Just because your experience matches those listed in Table 2.1 as anxiety doesn't mean you will inevitably see it as a problem for you. If you are uncertain, answer the following questions:

- Does my anxiety help me deal effectively with the threat?
- Does my anxiety motivate me in any way?

If you have answered 'yes' to either or both these questions, you may be reluctant to target your anxiety for change. Read the following section with an open mind and then answer two different questions.

Commit to concern as a productive alternative to anxiety

In any self-change venture, you need a clear alternative to the problem you wish to change; otherwise you'll be in a 'change vacuum', where you know what you don't want to feel but don't know what it would be healthy for you to feel instead. In RECBT, we argue that when you face (or think you face) a threat, the healthy alternative to feeling anxious about the threat is to feel concerned about it. Table 2.1 lists the behavioural and thinking consequences of RBs about threat associated with concern. If you see that these consequences will help you deal effectively with threat, you're ready to commit yourself to feeling concerned rather than anxious about threat.

If you're ambivalent about targeting anxiety as a problem to change in the previous section, answer the following while consulting the relevant sections of Table 2.1:

- Will anxiety or concern help me deal more effectively with the threat?
- Which is the more effective motivator: anxiety or concern?

Hopefully, if you were ambivalent about targeting your anxiety for change, you are now ready to do so and to work towards feeling concerned rather than anxious about threat.

Identify your threat

If you have a problem with anxiety, you may well experience this deadly emotion in situations where you infer the presence of a threat to some aspect of your personal domain. In this chapter your personal domain consists of:

- the ego realm where you infer the presence of threats to your self-esteem (see p. 15); and
- the non-ego realm where you infer the presence of threats to your sense of comfort, broadly defined (see p. 15).

Such threats can exist in both realms. To identify your threat, ask yourself, for example,

- What was I most anxious about in the situation I was in?
- What did I find most threatening in the situation I was in?

Use the 'magic question' technique

If you still have difficulty identifying your threat, use the 'magic question' technique:

- Focus on the situation in which you're anxious.
- Without changing the situation, ask yourself: 'What one thing would eliminate or significantly reduce my anxiety?'
- The opposite is what you're most anxious about.

Here is how Jeremy used this technique:

- I felt anxious in the tutorial room where six other students and the tutor were present.
- If I didn't say something stupid in the situation, I wouldn't be anxious.
- I'm most anxious about saying something stupid in the tutorial situation.

Identify the IBs underpinning your anxiety and the RBs underpinning concern

The RECBT model argues that threats to your personal domain don't make you anxious. Rather, you make yourself anxious by holding IBs (at 'B') about these threats, and if you hold RBs (also at 'B') about them instead, you will feel concerned but not anxious.

Consequently, you need to identify your IBs about your threat at 'A' and the rational alternatives to these IBs. I recommend doing the latter so you can derive hope that you can see an alternative to the main determining factor of your anxiety.

In identifying your IBs and alternative RBs, determine whether your anxiety is ego-related, involving a threat to your self-esteem, or non-ego-related, involving a threat to your sense of comfort, broadly defined, and not involving a threat to your self-esteem. Then do the following.

Ego anxiety

If your anxiety is ego-related, take your threat to your self-esteem; identify your rigid belief and self-depreciation belief about this threat; then identify their rational alternatives, i.e. your flexible belief and your unconditional self-acceptance belief.

Non-ego anxiety

If your anxiety is non-ego-related, take your threat to your sense of comfort, broadly defined; identify your rigid belief and either your awfulizing belief or discomfort intolerance belief about this threat; then identify their rational alternatives, i.e. your flexible belief and either your non-awfulizing belief or your discomfort tolerance belief.

Acknowledge the 'B–C' connection

Before proceeding to question these beliefs, acknowledge the connection between your IBs (at 'B') and your anxiety (at 'C') and between your RBs (also at 'B') and feelings of concern (at 'E') that you are aiming to experience in response to the threat (at 'A').

Question your beliefs

The purpose of the questioning process is for you to see clearly that your IBs are irrational (i.e. false, illogical and largely unhelpful) and that your alternative RBs are rational (i.e. true, logical and largely helpful). To enable you to get the most out of the questioning process, begin by questioning your rigid belief and flexible belief together. Ask yourself:

1 Which of these beliefs is true and which is false?
2 Which of these beliefs is logical and which is illogical?
3 Which of these beliefs is largely helpful and which is largely unhelpful?

Provide reasons for your answers. Appendix 2 gives suggestions concerning arguments on this issue. You should tailor your arguments to the content of your beliefs.

- If your anxiety is ego-based, take your self-depreciation belief and unconditional self-acceptance belief and question them by asking the same three questions as above. Provide reasons for your answers. Appendix 3 gives suggestions concerning arguments on this issue, which should be tailored to the content of your beliefs.
- If your anxiety is non-ego-based, take your awfulizing belief and non-awfulizing belief, or your discomfort intolerance belief and discomfort tolerance belief, and question the relevant pairing by asking the same three questions as above, giving reasons for your answers. Appendices 4 and 5 give suggestions concerning arguments on this issue, which should be tailored to the content of your beliefs.

At the end of this questioning process you should understand why your IBs are irrational and why the rational alternatives to these beliefs are rational. You should be able to commit yourself to act and think in ways consistent with your RBs to enable you to deal effectively with threats to your personal domain about which you made yourself anxious.

Face your threat in imagery

Hopefully you have made a commitment to act on your RBs (i.e. flexible belief and relevant non-extreme belief). Assuming you have, your basic task is to face your threat and learn to think rationally about it without using safety-seeking measures, withdrawing from life.

Up until now you have worked at a general level with respect to the threats you're anxious about, the IBs that account for this anxiety and their alternative RBs. However, when you apply your RBs in dealing with threat, bear in mind that since you make yourself anxious about specific threats (actual or imagined), you should deal with these specific threats by rehearsing specific variants of your general RBs.

While the best way to do this is in specific situations in which you infer threat, you may derive benefit by using imagery first. If so:

- Imagine a specific situation in which you felt or may feel anxious. Focus on your threat.
- See yourself facing the threat while rehearsing a specific RB relevant to the situation, but without using safety-seeking measures (behaviour or thinking). While doing so, try to make yourself feel concerned but not anxious.
- See yourself getting on with your life.
- Recognize that some of your post-belief thinking may be distorted. Respond without getting bogged down doing so. Accept the presence of any remaining distorted thoughts without engaging with them.
- Repeat the above steps until you feel sufficiently ready to put this sequence into practice in your life.

Face situations where you infer the presence of threat duly prepared but without using safety-seeking measures

Your work hitherto should be regarded as the foundation for the main ingredient in dealing effectively with your anxiety, i.e. facing your threat in reality without using safety-seeking measures.

You are prepared even though you may not feel it

If you have followed the previous steps, you're prepared to face your threat. Thus:

- You have equipped yourself with the RBs necessary to hold while facing the situations where you infer the presence of threat.
- You have identified safety-seeking measures to keep yourself safe from threat so you don't use them when facing threat-related situations.
- You understand the threat-exaggerating thoughts you have while anxious, so you can later learn to accept such thoughts without engaging with them.
- You have practised facing your threat in imagery.

Thus you are prepared to face your threat even though you may not feel prepared to face it. This is perfectly understandable, and as long as you don't believe you have to feel prepared before facing your threat you're now 'good to go'. The following are the steps you need to take to benefit from the RECBT approach to facing threat.

Take the following steps in facing threat

1 Choose a specific situation in which the threat is likely to occur and about which you would ordinarily feel anxious. Choose a situation which isn't too easy or difficult for you.
2 Make a plan of how you'll deal with the threat; resolve not to use any behavioural safety-seeking measures even if you feel the urge to do so.
3 Rehearse a specific version of your general RBs before entering the situation so you face your threat in a rational frame of mind. Moreover, it would be useful to develop a shorthand version of your specific RB to use while in the situation.
4 Enter the situation, focusing on what you find most threatening, and accept that you're likely to be uncomfortable doing so. Don't take any safety-seeking measures and take action as previously planned. React to any consequences from a rational frame of mind if you can. Accept the presence of thoughts designed to keep you safe; neither engage with them nor try to eliminate them.
5 Recognize that even though you've got yourself into a rational frame of mind, some of your thinking may still be distorted and unrealistic; some may be realistic and balanced. Accept the presence of the former and don't engage with it. Engage with the latter without using it to reassure yourself.

Capitalize on what you have learned and generalize your learning

Having faced your threat and dealt with it as best you can, it's important to reflect on what you did and what you have learned. In particular, if you were able to face your threat, rehearse your specific RBs and take constructive action. Ask yourself how you can capitalize on your achievement. Generalize your learning to similar threats or different threats.

Deal with any problems facing your threat

If you experienced any problems facing your threat using the above steps, respond to the following:

- Did I face the threat? If not, why not?
- Did I rehearse my RBs before and while facing the threat? If not, why not?
- Did I execute my plan to face the threat? If not, why not?
- Did I use safety-seeking measures? If so, why?
- Did I engage with post-belief distorted thinking? If so, why?

Reflect on your experience. Put into practice what you have learned next time you face the threat.

Become less prone to anxiety

So far I have discussed how to deal with anxiety about specified threats. However, if you're particularly prone to anxiety (i.e. you experience anxiety frequently about a variety of threats), I suggest the following.

Accept yourself unconditionally for being anxiety-prone

If prone to anxiety, for whatever reason, you have an important choice to make at the outset: accept yourself unconditionally as a fallible human being with a proneness to experiencing anxiety or depreciate yourself for this proneness. Before making your choice, bear in mind that unconditional self-acceptance doesn't mean you must resign yourself to a lifetime of anxiety-proneness. It means you're a fallible human being, whether or not prone to anxiety. It doesn't indicate that you cannot work to become less anxiety-prone. Indeed, it helps you do this. If you depreciate yourself for being anxiety-prone, you not only have emotional disturbance stemming from anxiety-proneness but are disturbing yourself about this disturbance – you have two disturbances for the price of one. Accepting yourself unconditionally for your anxiety-proneness not only spares you this secondary disturbance but helps you focus on your proneness with the purpose of helping yourself become less prone.

My advice then is: choose to accept yourself unconditionally for being prone to anxiety.

Deal with anxiety about anxiety

People often make themselves anxious about their anxiety. This can be an example of ego disturbance or non-ego disturbance.

Anxiety about anxiety: ego disturbance

Seeing anxiety as a sign of weakness and condemning oneself for this weakness is an example of ego disturbance (where people disturb themselves about their ego or self). The resultant shame leads to trying to suppress anxiety from others and, indeed, from oneself. If this applies to you, you'll know that your attempts to suppress anxiety will only make you more, not less, anxious and more prone to this deadly emotion. The antidote is to accept yourself as a fallible human being with strengths and weaknesses, with anxiety as one of your weaknesses (if you see it as a weakness).

Anxiety about anxiety: non-ego disturbance

People may additionally have non-ego disturbance about their anxiety, serving to perpetuate their anxiety and making them more, not less, prone to this deadly emotion. If this applies to you, you may disturb yourself about your anxiety because it is painful (and you think you can't stand the pain) or because it represents loss of self-control and you demand that you must always be in control of yourself. In these cases it is important to show yourself that:

- you can tolerate the pain of anxiety although it is unpleasant;
- you don't always need self-control although you may desire it. This flexible attitude helps you see that if you begin to lose control when feeling anxious, you won't inevitably lose complete self-control!

Develop a healthy attitude towards threat-related uncertainty

If you are intolerant of uncertainty about threat, you will be predisposed to infer the existence of this threat in the absence of supporting evidence for its existence. This is because you believe you have to know you are safe from threat and don't have such certainty; you conclude that such a threat exists if you aren't sure that it doesn't. Your rigid belief leads you to think in black-and-white terms. Either you know the threat doesn't exist or it does. In this rigid way of looking at the world, there's no place for you not knowing that the threat doesn't exist. You thus train yourself unwittingly to infer the presence of threat whenever uncertainty or ambiguity exist in situations where threats may occur. Then you make yourself anxious about this inferred threat by holding a set of IBs about it.

To deal with this vulnerability to anxiety:

- Show yourself that you can tolerate uncertainty about threat and that you don't have to know you are safe from threat, although this state of affairs would be preferable.
- Just because you don't know you're safe from threat or that you're in an ambiguous situation, it doesn't follow that the threat is present. It is quite possible that the threat is absent when you're in a state of uncertainty or facing ambiguity.
- If the threat does exist, develop and implement a set of RBs about it.

Examine the accuracy of your inference of threat if necessary

If you have developed an RB about uncertainty but are still unsure whether your inference of threat is accurate or inaccurate, answer one or more of the following:

- How likely is it that the threat happened (or might happen)?
- Would an objective jury agree that the threat actually happened or might happen? If not, what would the jury's verdict be?

- Did I view (am I viewing) the threat realistically? If not, how could I have viewed (can I view) it more realistically?
- If I asked someone I could trust to give me an objective opinion about the truth or falsity of my inference about the threat, what would that person say to me and why? How would he or she encourage me to view the threat instead?
- If a friend told me she had faced (were facing or were about to face) the same situation as I faced and had made the same inference of threat, what would I say to her about the validity of her inference and why? How would I encourage her to view the threat instead?

Understand the thinking consequences of your IBs

When you hold a set of IBs about threat then, as discussed, a consequence is that your subsequent thinking is highly distorted and skewed to the negative.

If you don't understand how your mind works in this respect, you'll get caught up in your compelling distorted thoughts and regard them as representing reality; you will thus strive to protect yourself from what you regard as real negative events rather than seeing them as highly distorted thinking consequences of IBs you have created.

However, if you do understand this phenomenon and act on this understanding, you'll trace such thinking back to the IBs that spawned it and will do one of two things (or both):

- question these IBs;
- acknowledge the existence of such distorted thinking and go about your business while neither engaging with it nor trying to eliminate it. You will maintain this understanding no matter how compelling your distorted thoughts are.

Summary

You can make yourself less prone to anxiety by:

- accepting yourself unconditionally for being anxiety-prone;
- dealing effectively with your anxiety about anxiety;
- developing a healthy attitude towards uncertainty related to threat, allowing you to make realistic threat-related inferences at 'A';
- understanding that when you hold IBs about threat, you exaggerate the nature of this threat and its consequences. However, you won't engage with such thinking but trace it back to the IBs that spawned it, which you will challenge. You will then let any remnants of such thinking be, without engaging with it or trying to eliminate it.

In the next chapter I will deal with the deadly emotion known as depression.

3

Dealing with depression

Depression is a very prevalent emotional problem. As mentioned in Chapter 2, along with anxiety it is the most common problem for which people seek help. This chapter outlines the RECBT view of depression and its healthy alternative, sadness, before showing what you need to do to deal effectively with this deadly emotion.

Understanding depression[3]

This section discusses the RECBT view of what happens when you make yourself depressed and how to deal effectively with this deadly emotion, using RECBT's 'ABC' model where 'A' stands for 'adversity', 'B' for beliefs and 'C' for the consequences of these beliefs. However, I will use the order 'CAB' since it's best to start with features of depression at 'C'.

'C'

Chapter 1 explained that there are three main features of any emotional problem: feeling, behavioural and thinking. You're likely to feel depression in several ways. Common experiences include a black mood, distorted negative thoughts about yourself, life and the future, difficulties with sleep (you can't sleep, sleep too much or wake very early), difficulties with eating (loss of appetite or overeating), irritability, lack of concentration. In severe or clinical depression you may feel suicidal, in which case please see your doctor as a matter of urgency; do not use this book if you feel actively suicidal. These feelings tend to interfere with thinking clearly about the adversity you have suffered (or think you have suffered) about which you feel depressed, and also tend to impede constructive action.

---

3 In this chapter, I'm talking about non-clinical depression. Clinical depression is characterized by a number of biological features such as insomnia, loss of appetite, loss of libido and thoughts of suicide. If you think you may be clinically depressed, consult your GP in the first instance.

Table 3.1 Depression vs sadness

Adversity	• You have experienced a loss from the sociotropic and/or autonomous realms of your personal domain.	
	• You have experienced failure within the sociotropic and/or autonomous realms of your personal domain.	
	• You or others have experienced an undeserved plight.	
Belief	*IRRATIONAL*	*RATIONAL*
Emotion	*Depression*	*Sadness*
Behaviour	• You become overly dependent on and seek to cling to others (particularly in sociotropic depression).	• You seek out reinforcements after a period of mourning (particularly when your inferential theme is loss).
	• You bemoan your fate or that of others to anyone who will listen (particularly in pity-based depression).	• You create an environment inconsistent with depressed feelings.
	• You create an environment consistent with your depressed feelings.	• You express your feelings about the loss, failure or undeserved plight and talk in a non-complaining way about these feelings to significant others.
	• You attempt to terminate feelings of depression in self-destructive ways.	
Subsequent thinking	• You see only negative aspects of the loss, failure or undeserved plight.	• You are able to recognize both negative and positive aspects of the loss or failure.
	• You think of other losses, failures and undeserved plights that you (and in the case of the latter, others) have experienced.	• You think you are able to help yourself.
	• You think you are unable to help yourself (helplessness).	• You look to the future with hope.
	• You only see pain and blackness in the future (hopelessness).	
	• You see yourself being totally dependent on others (in autonomous depression).	
	• You see yourself as being disconnected from others (in sociotropic depression).	
	• You see the world as full of undeservedness and unfairness (in plight-based depression).	
	• You tend to ruminate concerning the source of your depression and its consequences.	

Behaviour associated with depression

When depressed, you tend to act in several ways, outlined in Table 3.1.

Thinking associated with depression

When depressed, you tend to think about depression-related adversity in ways influenced by the irrational beliefs (IBs) you hold about such adversity. This type of thinking is known as cognitive distortions in CBT and is generally highly distorted in nature and skewed to the negative. I list and illustrate the main forms of cognitive distortions in Appendix 1, highlighting those particularly prevalent in depression in Table 3.1.

'A'

Chapter 1 explained that 'A' stands for adversity: what you're most disturbed about with respect to your personal domain. When depressed, three realms of your personal domain are implicated in your depression:

- *Autonomous realm* Here you value freedom from influence, freedom from constraint, freedom to determine your fate, independence, self-control and effective functioning.
- *Sociotropic realm* Here you value your relationships and connections with people, being loved, approved, cared for by them, being able to rely on them and to look after them.
- *Deservingness realm* Here you value yourself and others being treated fairly by the world.

The major inference themes in depression

When you experience depression you tend to make one or more inferences related to these three realms of your personal domain.

Loss   Here you infer that you have lost something important from the autonomous and/or sociotropic realms of your personal domain.

Failure   Here you infer that you have experienced a failure within the autonomous and/or sociotropic realms of your personal domain.

Undeserved plight   Here you infer that you and/or others have experienced an undeserved plight.[4]

'B'

As Chapter 1 explained, beliefs are at the heart of the RECBT model of the emotions. Loss/failure/undeserved plight, within salient realms

---

4 When I discuss undeserved plight in this chapter, I'm referring to such a plight that can befall you and/or others.

of your personal domain, on their own do not explain your depressed response, since you can make the same inferences as listed above and be sad, but not depressed. To feel depressed when you infer the presence of loss/failure/undeserved plight, you have to hold a set of IBs.

IBs about loss/failure/undeserved plight

The RECBT model of depression is that you feel depressed about losses/ failures/undeserved plights within salient realms of your personal domain when you hold IBs about these inferences.[5] These beliefs are rigid and extreme. Please note:

- rigid beliefs are common to both ego depression and non-ego depression;
- self-depreciation beliefs are the main extreme beliefs in ego depression;
- awfulizing beliefs or discomfort intolerance beliefs are the main extreme beliefs in non-ego depression.

Understanding sadness

As Chapter 1 explained, when you face a negative event it is healthy to experience a negative emotion that helps you deal effectively with the negative event you face. This section discusses the RECBT view of sadness as the healthy alternative to depression, again using the 'CABDE' order of the 'ABCDE' framework.

'C'

As explained above, there are three main features of depression: feeling, behavioural, thinking. The same is true when you're sad but not depressed. When sad, you may feel low (rather than experiencing a black mood) and lack energy, but you can still function in daily life. These feelings will encourage you to think clearly about the loss/failure/ undeserved plight you have (or think you have) experienced and motivate you to take constructive action.

Behaviour associated with sadness

When you're sad but not depressed, you're motivated to face and deal with loss/failure/undeserved plight. Table 3.1 outlines the major ways you feel like acting when sad.

---

5 Remember that the important point here is that you think you've lost something, failed at something or experienced an undeserved plight, whether you have or not.

Thinking associated with sadness

When you're sad but not depressed, you tend to think in ways designed to help you face and deal effectively with depression-related adversities (see Table 3.1). The dominant feature of thinking associated with sadness is that it is realistic and optimistic.

'A'

When you're sad, your feelings are about the same things about which you felt depressed (loss/failure/undeserved plight – see Table 3.1).

'B'

When you're sad but not depressed about loss/failure/undeserved plight, the beliefs you hold about these adversities are rational.

Rational beliefs about loss/failure/undeserved plight

The RECBT model of sadness is to feel sad but not depressed about losses/failures/undeserved plights within salient realms of your personal domain when you hold rational beliefs (RBs) about these adversities. These beliefs are flexible and non-extreme. Please note:

- Flexible beliefs are common to both ego sadness and non-ego sadness.
- Unconditional self-acceptance beliefs are the main non-extreme beliefs in ego sadness.
- Non-awfulizing beliefs or discomfort tolerance beliefs are the main non-extreme beliefs in non-ego sadness.

Dealing with depression

Since you make yourself depressed about loss/failure/undeserved plight, your goal is to make yourself sad but not depressed about the same adversities. That's why I will encourage you to assume temporarily that your inferences of loss/failure/undeserved plight at 'A' are correct. Once you're sad but not depressed, you'll be in a sufficiently rational frame of mind to examine your loss/failure/undeserved plight inferences. If you're depressed about these adversities you won't be objective enough while examining your inferences. Later, I will also explain why you are prone to inferring the existence of depression-related inferences in ambiguous situations and will help you become less prone.

Ensure that you're feeling depressed and it's a problem for you

Before doing anything to try to change depression feelings, ensure that you're depressed and see that depression is a problem for you. Otherwise, you'll resist your own efforts to help yourself.

Are you depressed?

People use the term 'depressed' loosely; if you say you're depressed, you may or may not be experiencing the deadly version of this emotion. Determine whether you're experiencing the deadly version by consulting the behavioural and thinking consequences of both IBs and RBs about loss/failure/undeserved plight. The more your behaviour and thinking match those listed in Table 3.1 as consequences of IBs, the more likely you are (or were) to be depressed rather than sad. Conversely, the more your behaviour and thinking match those listed as consequences of RBs, the more likely you are (or were) to be sad rather than depressed.

Is depression a problem for you?

Assuming you've determined you're depressed rather than sad, now determine whether you consider your depression is a problem you want to change. Just because your experience matches those listed in Table 3.1 as depression doesn't mean you'll inevitably see it's a problem for you.

If you're uncertain if depression is a problem for you, answer the following:

- Does my depression help me deal effectively with loss/failure/undeserved plight?
- Does my depression motivate me in any way?

If you've answered 'yes' to either or both questions, you may be reluctant to target your depression for change. I suggest you read the following section with an open mind and then answer two different questions.

Commit to sadness as a productive alternative to depression

In any self-change venture, you need clear alternatives to problems you wish to change. Otherwise you'll be in a 'change vacuum', where you know what you don't want to feel but don't know what it would be healthy for you to feel instead. RECBT argues that when you've experienced (or think you've experienced) a loss/failure/undeserved plight, the healthy alternative to feeling depressed about these depression-related adversities is to feel concerned about them. Table 3.1 lists the behavioural and thinking consequences of RBs about loss/failure/undeserved plight associated with sadness. If you see that these consequences help you deal effectively with loss/failure/undeserved plight, then you're ready to commit yourself to feeling sad rather than depressed about these inferences or facts at 'A'.

For those ambivalent about targeting depression as a problem to change in the previous section, answer the following questions while consulting the relevant sections of Table 3.1:

- Will depression or sadness help me deal more effectively with loss/failure/undeserved plight?
- Which is the more effective motivator: depression or sadness?

Hopefully, if you were ambivalent about targeting your depression for change you're now ready to do so and to work towards feeling sad rather than depressed about loss/failure/undeserved plight.

Become active

As Table 3.1 indicates, when depressed you tend to become inactive; this can lead to more negative thinking, leading in turn to decreased activity. The sooner you can go against your tendency to become inactive, the better. If your inactivity hasn't become ingrained, increased activity helps in two ways. First, it can be an anti-depressant, particularly if it involves exercise. Running has been shown to be an effective antidote to mild depression. Second, increased activity facilitates greater concentration on the psychological work that the remaining steps call for.

However, what can you do if you've become very inactive and don't think you can become more active or think that, if you did, it wouldn't make any difference? First, you need to see resistance to becoming active as depressed thinking stemming from the IBs that led to your depression in the first place. Rather than responding to it, you should test these thoughts out behaviourally. Thus, if you think you can't become active, test it out by seeing if you can walk to the end of the road. If you can, take another step and proceed, bit by bit, until you've become more active. At that point you can judge whether or not becoming more active has had any impact on your mood, which it certainly will.

Having improved your mood to the point that you can concentrate, you're ready to resume the psychological work necessary to deal effectively with your depression.

Identify your depression-related theme

If you have a problem with depression, you're likely to experience this deadly emotion in situations where you infer you've failed in the autonomous or sociotropic realms of your personal domain or when you think that you or others have experienced an undeserved plight. Your depression may be ego-based or non-ego-based.

Use the 'magic question' technique

If you still cannot identify your depression-related theme, use the 'magic question' technique:

- Focus on the situation in which you were depressed.

- Without changing the situation, ask yourself: 'What one thing would eliminate or significantly reduce my depression?'
- The opposite is what you're most depressed about.

Here's how Lorna used this technique:

- I felt depressed when I learned my application to my preferred university was rejected.
- If my freedom to do what I want was intact, I wouldn't be depressed.
- I'm most depressed about my freedom to do what I want being curtailed.

Identify the IBs underpinning your depression and the rational alternatives underpinning sadness

The RECBT model argues that loss/failure/undeserved plights don't make you depressed. Rather, you make yourself depressed by holding IBs (at 'B') about these adversities and if you hold RBs (also at 'B') about them instead, then you'll feel sad but not depressed.

Consequently, you should identify your IBs about your loss/failure/ undeserved plight at 'A' and the rational alternatives to these IBs. I recommend the latter so you can derive hope that you can see there's an alternative to the main determining factor of your depression.

In identifying your IBs and alternative RBs, determine whether your depression is ego-related, with implications for your self-esteem, or non-ego-related, with implications for your sense of comfort, broadly defined, but not for your self-esteem. Then do the following.

Ego depression

If your depression is ego-related, identify your rigid belief and self-depreciation belief about loss or failure. Then identify their rational alternatives, i.e. your flexible belief and unconditional self-acceptance belief.

Non-ego depression

If your depression is non-ego-related, identify your rigid belief and either your awfulizing belief or discomfort intolerance belief about loss/ failure/undeserved plight. Then identify their rational alternatives, i.e. your flexible belief and either your non-awfulizing belief or discomfort tolerance belief.

Acknowledge the 'B–C' connection

Before proceeding to question these beliefs, acknowledge the connection between your IBs (at 'B') and depression (at 'C') and between your RBs (at 'B') and feelings of sadness (at 'E') that you're aiming to experience in response to the loss/failure/undeserved plight (at 'A').

Question your beliefs

You're now ready to question your beliefs to see clearly that your IBs are irrational (i.e. false, illogical and largely unhelpful) and that your alternative RBs are rational (i.e. true, logical and largely helpful). To enable you to get the most out of this process:

- Begin by questioning your rigid belief and flexible belief together. Ask yourself:
  - Which of these beliefs is true? Which is false?
  - Which of these beliefs is logical? Which is illogical?
  - Which of these beliefs is largely helpful? Which is largely unhelpful?

  Provide reasons for your answers. See Appendix 2 for suggestions concerning arguments on this issue. You'll need to tailor your arguments to the content of your beliefs.

- If your depression is ego-based, take your self-depreciation belief and unconditional self-acceptance belief and question them by asking the same three questions as above. Again provide reasons for your answers. See Appendix 3 for suggestions concerning arguments on this issue, which have to be tailored to the content of your beliefs.

- If your depression is non-ego-based, either take your awfulizing belief and non-awfulizing belief or your discomfort intolerance belief and discomfort tolerance belief and question the relevant pairing by asking the same three questions as above, providing reasons for your answers. See Appendices 4 and 5 for suggestions concerning arguments on this issue, which have to be tailored to the content of your beliefs.

Having completed this process you should understand why your IBs are irrational and why the rational alternatives to these beliefs are rational, and will be in a position to commit yourself to act and think in ways consistent with your RBs to enable you to deal effectively with the loss/failure/undeserved plight about which you made yourself depressed.

Face your loss/failure/undeserved plight in imagery

Assuming you've committed to act on your RBs (flexible belief and relevant non-extreme belief), you must face up to your loss/failure/undeserved plight and learn to think rationally about it without withdrawing from life.

Until now you've worked generally in regard to losses/failures/undeserved plights you're depressed about, the general IBs that account for this depression and their alternative general RBs. However, to apply these general RBs in dealing with loss/failure/undeserved plight, you must remember that since you make yourself depressed about specific losses/

failures/undeserved plights (actual or imagined), you should deal with these specific losses by rehearsing specific variants of your general RBs.

The best way to do this is in specific situations in which you infer loss/failure/undeserved plight, but you may benefit by first using imagery as follows:

1 Imagine a specific situation in which you could feel depressed; focus on your loss/failure/undeserved plight.
2 Picture yourself facing the loss/failure/undeserved plight while rehearsing a specific and relevant RB. Try to make yourself feel sad but not depressed.
3 Imagine yourself getting on with your life after an appropriate period of mourning and recognize that it's healthy to feel sad even well after the event. Your sadness doesn't prevent you from reconnecting with life and following your goals.
4 Recognize that some of your post-belief thinking may be distorted. Respond without getting bogged down doing so. Accept the presence of any remaining distorted thoughts without engaging with them.
5 Repeat these steps until you feel ready to put this sequence into practice in your life.

Face your loss/failure/undeserved plight in reality

Even if you haven't used imagery as a preparatory step, take the following steps when you face situations reminding you of your loss/failure/undeserved plight.

- Choose a specific situation in which you'll be reminded of your loss/failure/undeserved plight and about which you would ordinarily feel depressed.
- Rehearse a specific version of your general RBs before entering the situation so you can face your loss/failure/undeserved plight while in a rational frame of mind. Develop a shorthand version of your specific RB to use while in the situation.
- Enter the situation, accepting that you're likely to be uncomfortable doing so. React to any consequences rationally if you can.
- Even if you've got yourself into a rational frame of mind, accept that some of your thinking may be distorted and unrealistic; some may be realistic and balanced. Accept the former's presence and don't engage with it; engage with the latter without using it to reassure yourself.

Capitalize on what you have learned and generalize your learning

When you've faced your loss/failure/undeserved plight and dealt with it as best you could, reflect on what you did and what you learned. In particular, if you were able to face your loss/failure/undeserved plight, rehearse your specific RBs and take constructive action, then ask yourself how you can capitalize on what you achieved. And generalize your learning to both similar and different losses/failures/undeserved plights.

Deal with any problems facing loss/failure/undeserved plight

If you experienced problems facing loss/failure/undeserved plight using the above steps, answer the following:

- Did I face the loss/failure/undeserved plight? If not, why not?
- Did I rehearse my RBs before and during facing the adversity? If not, why not?
- Did I execute my plan to face the adversity? If not, why not?
- Did I engage with post-belief distorted thinking? If so, why?

Reflect on your experience and put into practice what you learned the next time you face loss/failure/undeserved plight.

Become less depression-prone

So far I've discussed how you can help yourself deal with depression about specified loss/failure/undeserved plight. However, if you're particularly depression-prone (i.e. experience depression frequently about a variety of losses/failures/undeserved plights), do the following.

Accept yourself unconditionally for being depression-prone

If depression-prone for whatever reason, you have an important choice to make at the outset: you can accept yourself unconditionally as a fallible human being, prone to experiencing depression, or you can depreciate yourself for this proneness. Before making your choice, please remember that unconditional self-acceptance doesn't mean you need to resign yourself to a lifetime of depression-proneness. It means you're a fallible human being whether or not you're depression-prone. It doesn't indicate that you cannot work to become less depression-prone. Indeed, it helps you do this. If you depreciate yourself for being depression-prone, you not only have emotional disturbance stemming from depression-proneness, you're disturbing yourself about this disturbance: you have two disturbances for the price of one. So accepting yourself unconditionally for being depression-prone not only spares you this secondary disturbance, it helps you focus on your proneness with the purpose of helping you become less prone.

My advice then is: choose to accept yourself unconditionally for being depression-prone.

Develop a healthy attitude towards ambiguity about loss/ failure/undeserved plight

A main reason why you may be vulnerable to depression is that you may easily infer that you've experienced a loss/failure/undeserved plight in the face of ambiguity and bring a set of IBs to these inferences. But why make such inferences so easily? I consider the reason is that you are intolerant of ambiguity about loss/failure/undeserved plight. Because you believe you have to know whether or not you have experienced a loss/failure/undeserved plight, when things aren't so clear-cut you conclude that you've experienced one of these adversities because you cannot convince yourself you haven't. Your rigid belief leads you to think in black-and-white terms. Either you know you haven't experienced a loss/failure/undeserved plight or you have experienced it. In this rigid way of looking at the world, there's no place for ambiguity or uncertainty related to loss/failure/undeserved plight. In this way you train yourself, unwittingly, to infer the presence of loss/failure/undeserved plight whenever uncertainty or ambiguity exists in situations where such adversities may be present. Then, as mentioned above, you make yourself depressed about loss/failure/undeserved plight by holding a set of IBs about it.

To deal with this vulnerability to depression, do the following:

- Show yourself you can tolerate uncertainty and ambiguity about the possible presence of loss/failure/undeserved plight and that you don't have to have clarity, although this state of affairs would be preferable.
- Just because you're not clear about the presence of loss/failure/undeserved plight, it doesn't follow that such adversities are present. It's quite possible that you haven't experienced one of these adversities when you're in a state of uncertainty or facing ambiguity.
- If you have experienced loss/failure/undeserved plight, develop and implement a set of RBs about it.

How to examine the accuracy of your inference of loss/failure/ undeserved plight if necessary

If you're still unsure whether you've experienced a loss/failure/undeserved plight, answer one or more of the following questions (focusing on failure to exemplify the points made):

- How valid is my conclusion that I failed?
- Would an objective jury agree that I failed? If not, what would their verdict be?
- Is my conclusion that I failed realistic? If not, what is a more realistic conclusion?

- If I asked someone I could trust to give me an objective opinion about my conclusion that I failed, what would that person say to me and why? What conclusion would he or she encourage me to make instead?
- If a friend told me he had made the same conclusion that he had failed, what would I say to him about the validity of his conclusion and why? What conclusion would I encourage him to make instead?

Dealing with emotional problems about depression

Meta-disturbance is literally disturbance about disturbance. It's important to assess carefully the nature of this meta-disturbance about depression before you can best deal with it.

Assessing emotional problems about depression

Again, the best way to start dealing with the assessment of any emotional problems you might have about depression is to ask yourself: 'How do I feel about being depressed?' The most common emotional problems people have about depression are: anxiety, depression, guilt, shame and unhealthy self-anger. I'll discuss only the second of these in this chapter, i.e. depression about depression, and refer you to the respective chapters on anxiety, guilt, shame and unhealthy anger for how to deal with these emotional problems as applied to depression.

Assessing depression about depression

When you're depressed about depression, it's clear that you think of your original depression as a loss/failure/undeserved plight. The most common inferences are:

- Depression means I have lost connection with people (in the sociotropic realm).
- Depression means I have to rely on others (in the autonomic realm).
- Depression is an additional undeserved burden I have to deal with (in the undeservingness realm).

Dealing with depression about depression

Unless you deal with your depression about depression (called meta-depression), you're unlikely to deal with your original depression, since your meta-depression will lead you to focus on themes about which you're likely to feel even more depressed. Thus, meta-depression (if you experience it) often has to be dealt with before dealing with your original depression.

As I've made clear in this book, it's important you develop and apply RBs about loss/failure/undeserved plight, while becoming more active and letting be (i.e. not engaging with or distracting yourself from) any remaining post-IB negative thoughts or images you may have. With these points in mind, here's how to deal with the three forms of depression about depression I've listed.

Dealing with the loss of connection with others

This is an issue you're more likely to have if your depression is in the sociotropic realm than if it is in the autonomous or undeservingness realms. To deal with it, first develop a set of RBs about the loss of connection with others (after questioning both your IBs and RBs as outlined in Appendices 2–5). These may be ego in nature (e.g. 'I'd prefer not to lose connection with others, but that doesn't mean it mustn't happen. If it does, that's unfortunate, but doesn't prove I'm unlovable. I'm an unrateable person, capable of being loved whether I'm connected to others or not') or non-ego in nature (e.g. 'I'd prefer not to lose connection with others, but that doesn't mean it mustn't happen. If it does, it's a struggle for me to put up with this uncomfortable situation, but I can tolerate it and it's worth it to me to do so'). Then, it's useful for you to develop a shorthand version of these RBs (e.g. 'Connection with others is good, but not necessary') and use this before seeking to reconnect with others and as you do so.

Dealing with relying on others

When you're depressed, you may lose some autonomy and be forced to rely on others. This is a particular problem for those who are rigid about having autonomy. If you're likely to make yourself depressed about having to rely on others, first develop a set of RBs about having to rely on others (after questioning both your IBs and RBs as outlined in Appendices 2–5). These may be ego in nature (e.g. 'I'd prefer not to rely on others, but I don't always have to have this wish fulfilled. If I do have to rely on others this doesn't prove I'm a weak person. I'm a fallible person whose worth does not change if I have to rely on others') or non-ego in nature (e.g. 'I'd prefer not to rely on others, but I do not always have to have my wish fulfilled on this issue. If I do have to rely on others that's unfortunate, but it isn't terrible'). It's again useful to develop a shorthand version of these RBs (e.g. 'I'm fallible, not weak, if I have to rely on others') and use this before seeking help from others and as you do so.

Dealing with the additional burden of depression

The first step to dealing with this depression is to assume temporarily that depression is an additional burden. Then develop a set of RBs about having such an undeserved plight (after questioning both your IBs and RBs as outlined in Appendices 2–4). These are likely to be non-ego in nature (e.g. 'I'd prefer not to have this additional undeserved burden on me, but that doesn't mean I mustn't have it. It's unfortunate I have it, but not terrible and I'm not a poor person as a result. I'm a non-poor person in a poor situation'). Again it's useful to develop a shorthand version of this RB (e.g. 'Depression is poor, but I'm not') and use this before tackling your original depression.

Understand the thinking consequences of your IBs

When you hold a set of IBs about loss/failure/undeserved plight then, as already discussed, a consequence is that your subsequent thinking is highly distorted and skewed to the negative.

If you don't understand how your mind works in this respect, you'll get caught up in your compelling distorted thoughts, regard them as representing reality and strive to protect yourself from what you regard as real negative events rather than seeing them as highly distorted thinking consequences of IBs you have created.

However, if you do understand this phenomenon and act on this understanding, you'll trace such thinking back to the IBs that spawned it and will do one of two things (or both):

- you will question these IBs;
- you will acknowledge the existence of such distorted thinking and go about your business while neither engaging with it nor trying to eliminate it. You will maintain this understanding no matter how compelling your distorted thoughts are.

Summary

You can make yourself less depression-prone by:

- accepting yourself unconditionally for being depression-prone;
- dealing effectively with your emotional problems about depression;
- developing a healthy attitude towards uncertainty and ambiguity related to loss/failure/undeserved plight so that you make more realistic inferences about their presence at 'A';
- understanding that when you hold IBs about loss/failure/undeserved plight, you will exaggerate the nature of this and its consequences. However, you will not engage with such thinking but trace it back to the IBs that spawned it, which you will challenge. You will then let any remnants of such thinking be, again without engaging with it or trying to eliminate it.

In the next chapter, I deal with the deadly emotion known as guilt.

4

Dealing with guilt

Guilt is a deadly emotion that stops you from taking risks and leads you to act in ways where you end up feeling that your life isn't your own. While others may see you as virtuous, some may take advantage of you and you don't assert yourself to stop them. This chapter outlines the RECBT view of guilt and its healthy alternative, remorse, before showing what you need to do to deal effectively with this deadly emotion.

Understanding guilt

This section discusses the RECBT view of what happens when you make yourself guilty and how to deal effectively with this deadly emotion, using RECBT's 'ABC' model where 'A' stands for 'adversity', 'B' for beliefs and 'C' for the consequences of these beliefs. However, I will use the order 'CAB' since it's best to start with features of guilt at 'C'.

'C'

Chapter 1 explained that there are three main features of any emotional problem: feeling, behavioural and thinking. You're likely to feel guilt in several ways. If you focus on what you feel guilty about and depreciate yourself, you'll tend to experience depression-like symptoms such as being in a black mood and having difficulties sleeping (see Chapter 3, p. 26, for a list of depressive symptoms). If you're scared of retribution – divine or otherwise – you'll experience anxiety-like symptoms such as a general feeling of dread (see Chapter 2, p. 12, for a list of anxiety symptoms). These symptoms tend to interfere with thinking clearly about what you feel guilty about and also tend to impede constructive action.

Behaviour associated with guilt

When feeling guilty, you tend to act in several ways, outlined in Table 4.1. Some of these behaviours are designed to help you escape from the pain of guilt; others are more linked to your tendency to want to punish yourself. You may switch between these different behaviours even within a single episode of guilt.

Table 4.1 Guilt vs remorse

Adversity	• You have broken your moral code. • You have failed to live up to your moral code. • You have hurt someone's feelings.	
Belief	IRRATIONAL	RATIONAL
Emotion	Guilt	Remorse
Behaviour	• You escape from the unhealthy pain of guilt in self-defeating ways. • You beg forgiveness from the person you have wronged. • You promise unrealistically that you will not 'sin' again. • You punish yourself physically or by deprivation. • You defensively disclaim responsibility for wrongdoing. • You reject offers of forgiveness.	• You face up to the healthy pain that accompanies the realization that you have sinned. • You ask, but do not beg, for forgiveness. • You understand the reasons for your wrongdoing and act on your understanding. • You atone for the sin by taking a penalty. • You make appropriate amends. • You do not make excuses for your behaviour or enact other defensive behaviour. • You accept offers of forgiveness.
Subsequent thinking	• You conclude that you have definitely committed the sin. • You assume more personal responsibility than the situation warrants. • You assign far less responsibility to others than is warranted. • You dismiss possible mitigating factors for your behaviour. • You only see your behaviour in a guilt-related context and fail to put it into an overall context. • You think that you will receive retribution.	• You take into account all relevant data when judging whether or not you have 'sinned'. • You assume an appropriate level of personal responsibility. • You assign an appropriate level of responsibility to others. • You take into account mitigating factors. • You put your behaviour into an overall context. • You think you may be penalized rather than receive retribution.

Thinking associated with guilt

When feeling guilt, you tend to think in ways that exaggerate the 'badness' of what you've done, which you don't contextualize, and you take far more responsibility than warranted (see Table 4.1 for a full list of thinking that accompanies guilt).

'A'

Chapter 1 explained that 'A' stands for adversity: what you're most disturbed about with respect to your personal domain. When feeling guilt, the inferences you make (what you feel guilty about) have to do with the moral realm of your personal domain. Thus:

- you think you've broken your moral code (i.e. done the wrong thing);
- you think you've failed to live up to your moral code (i.e. failed to do the right thing);
- you think you've hurt someone's feelings.

As with all deadly emotions, when you feel guilty you think your inferences are facts.

'B'

As Chapter 1 explained, beliefs are at the heart of the RECBT model of the emotions. When you make one or more of the three guilt-related inferences listed, these inferences, on their own, don't explain your guilt, since, as I'll show, it's possible and desirable to feel remorse when you have done the wrong thing, have failed to do the right thing or have hurt someone's feelings. Chapter 1 indicated that you can hold a set of IBs or RBs about adversity.

IBs about guilt-related inferences

The RECBT model of guilt is that you feel guilty about breaching your moral code or hurting someone's feelings when you hold IBs about these guilt-related inferences. These beliefs are rigid and extreme in that you depreciate yourself as bad.

Understanding remorse

As Chapter 1 explained, when you face a negative event it's healthy to experience a negative emotion that helps you deal effectively with the negative event you face. This section discusses the RECBT view of remorse as the healthy alternative to guilt, again using the 'CABDE' order of the 'ABCDE' framework.

'C'

As explained above, there are three main features of guilt: feeling, behavioural and thinking. The same is true when you're feeling remorse but not guilt. When remorseful, you may feel symptoms related to concern (see p. 16) and sadness (see p. 29), but not those related to anxiety (see p. 12) and depression (see p. 26). These feelings will encourage you to think clearly about your guilt-related inference and motivate you to take constructive action.

Behaviour associated with remorse

When feeling remorse but not guilt, you're motivated to face what you feel remorseful about and deal with it. Table 4.1 outlines the major ways you feel like acting when remorseful.

Thinking associated with remorse

When feeling remorse but not guilt, you tend to think in ways designed to help you face and deal effectively with what you feel remorseful about. Such thinking also takes into account contextual factors of your original behaviour and reflects your taking the appropriate amount of responsibility (see Table 4.1).

'A'

When you're remorseful but not guilty, the themes about which you feel remorse are the same as those about which you feel guilt, namely: breaching your moral code or hurting someone's feelings (see Table 4.1).

'B'

When you feel remorse but not guilt about breaching your moral code or hurting someone's feelings, you do so because the beliefs you hold about these inferences are rational.

RBs about breaching your moral code or hurting someone's feelings

The RECBT model of remorse is to feel remorse but not guilt about breaching your moral code or hurting someone's feelings when you hold RBs about these inferences. These beliefs are flexible and non-extreme in that you accept yourself as fallible.

How to deal with guilt

Since you make yourself guilty about breaching your moral code or hurting someone's feelings, your goal is to make yourself remorseful but not guilty about these inferences. That's why I'll encourage you to assume temporarily that your inferences that you have breached your moral code or hurt someone's feelings at 'A' are correct. Once you're remorseful rather than guilty, you'll be in a sufficiently rational frame of mind to examine your guilt-related inferences. If you're guilty about them you won't be objective enough while examining your inferences. Later, I'll explain why you're prone to thinking you have breached your moral code or hurt someone's feelings in ambiguous situations and will help you become less prone.

Ensure that you're feeling guilt and it's a problem for you

Before doing anything to try to change guilty feelings, ensure that you're feeling guilt and that you see that guilt is a problem for you. Otherwise, you'll resist your own efforts to help yourself.

Are you feeling guilt?

People use the term 'guilt' loosely; if you say you feel guilty, you may or may not be experiencing the deadly version of this emotion. Determine whether you're experiencing the deadly version by consulting the behavioural and thinking consequences of both IBs and RBs about having breached your moral code or hurt someone's feelings. The more your behaviour and thinking match those listed in Table 4.1 as consequences of IBs, the more likely you are (or were) feeling guilty rather than remorseful. Conversely, the more your behaviour and thinking match those listed as consequences of RBs, the more likely you are (or were) feeling remorse rather than guilt.

Is guilt a problem for you?

Assuming you've determined that you experienced guilt rather than remorse, now determine whether or not you consider your guilt is a problem you want to change. Just because your experience matches those listed in Table 4.1 as guilt doesn't mean you'll inevitably see it's a problem for you.

If you're uncertain whether guilt is a problem for you, answer the following:

- Does my guilt help me deal effectively with breaching my moral code or hurting someone's feelings?
- Does my guilt help me contextualize what I did and/or take appropriate responsibility for my behaviour?

If you've answered 'yes' to either or both questions, you may be reluctant to target your guilt for change. I suggest you read the following section with an open mind and then answer two different questions.

Commit to remorse as a productive alternative to guilt

In any self-change venture, you need clear alternatives to problems you wish to change. Otherwise you'll be in a 'change vacuum', where you know what you don't want to feel but don't know what it would be healthy for you to feel instead. RECBT argues that when you face (or think you're facing) a situation where you've breached your moral code or hurt someone's feelings, the healthy alternative to feeling guilt is to feel remorseful. Table 4.1 lists the behavioural and thinking consequences of RBs about breaching your moral code or hurting someone's feelings associated with remorse. If you see that these consequences help you deal effectively with breaching your moral code or hurting someone's feelings, then you're ready to commit yourself to feeling remorse rather than guilt about these inferences.

For those ambivalent about targeting guilt as a problem to change in the previous section, answer the following questions while consulting the relevant sections of Table 4.1:

- Will guilt or remorse help me deal more effectively with breaching my moral code or hurting someone's feelings?
- Which will help me contextualize my behaviour and allow me to take appropriate responsibility for my behaviour: guilt or remorse?

Hopefully, if you were ambivalent about targeting your guilt for change, you're now ready to do so and to work towards feeling remorseful rather than guilty about breaching your moral code or hurting someone's feelings.

Identify what you are most guilty about

If you have a problem with guilt, you're likely to experience this deadly emotion in situations where you infer that:

- you've broken your moral code;
- you've failed to live up to your moral code;
- you've hurt someone's feelings.

To identify your guilt-related inference, ask yourself, regarding when you felt guilt:

- What did I feel most guilty about in the situation I was in?
- When I felt guilt:
  - what did I do in the situation that I thought was wrong?
  - what did I fail to do in the situation that would have been the right thing to do?
  - whose feelings did I think I hurt and how did I do this?

Use the 'magic question' technique

If you still cannot identify your guilt-related inference, use the 'magic question' technique:

- Focus on the situation in which you felt guilty.
- Without changing the situation, ask yourself: 'What one thing would eliminate or significantly reduce my guilt?'

- The opposite is what you're most guilty about.

Here's how Fay used this technique:

- I felt guilty when I learned that my friend had been robbed at the club.
- If I had warned her to take care of her possessions, I wouldn't have felt guilty.
- I'm most guilty about not warning her.

Identify the IBs underpinning your guilt and the rational alternatives underpinning remorse

The RECBT model argues that guilt-related inferences don't make you feel guilty. Rather, you make yourself feel guilty by holding IBs (at 'B') about these inferences and if you hold RBs (also at 'B') about them instead, then you'll feel remorse but not guilt.

Consequently, you should identify your IBs about your guilt-related inferences at 'A' and the rational alternatives to these IBs. I recommend the latter so you can derive hope that you can see there's an alternative to the main determining factor of your guilt.

In identifying your IBs, specify your rigid belief and extreme self-depreciation belief, and in identifying your alternative RBs, specify your flexible belief and non-extreme unconditional self-acceptance belief.

Acknowledge the 'B–C' connection

Before proceeding to question these beliefs, acknowledge the connection between your IBs (at 'B') and guilt (at 'C') and between your RBs (at 'B') and remorse feelings (at 'E') that you're aiming to experience in response to breaching your moral code or hurting someone's feelings (at 'A').

Question your beliefs

You're now ready to question your beliefs to see clearly that your IBs are irrational (i.e. false, illogical and largely unhelpful) and that your alternative RBs are rational (i.e. true, logical and largely helpful). To enable you to get the most out of this process:

- Begin by questioning your rigid belief and flexible belief together. Ask yourself:
  - Which of these beliefs is true? Which is false?
  - Which of these beliefs is logical? Which is illogical?
  - Which of these beliefs is largely helpful? Which is largely unhelpful?
  Provide reasons for your answers. See Appendix 2 for suggestions concerning arguments on this issue. You'll need to tailor your arguments to the content of your beliefs.
- Take your self-depreciation belief and unconditional self-acceptance belief and question them by asking the same three questions as

above. Again provide reasons for your answers. See Appendix 3 for suggestions concerning arguments on this issue, which have to be tailored to the content of your beliefs.

Having completed this process you should understand why your IBs are irrational and why the rational alternatives to these beliefs are rational, and will be in a position to commit yourself to act and think in ways consistent with your RBs to enable you to deal effectively with breaching your moral code or hurting someone's feelings, about which you made yourself feel guilty.

Take appropriate responsibility and understand your behaviour in context

Having questioned your beliefs and committed yourself to your RBs, look again at events about which you've made yourself guilty, this time rationally (i.e. using flexible and unconditional self-acceptance beliefs). This involves your taking responsibility for your behaviour, but recognizing that others have responsibility too. You also need to understand your behaviour in context by considering the factors involved in the situation. When you feel guilt, you see things in black and white, tending to take far too much responsibility and editing out the impact of external factors. In remorse, you recognize the complexity of the situation and that there are many influences on your behaviour.

Remorse helps you learn from situations in which you think you've breached your moral code or have hurt someone's feelings and to use this learning in future situations.

Face your guilt-related theme in imagery

Assuming you've committed to act on your RBs (flexible belief and unconditional self-acceptance belief), you must face up to doing the wrong thing, failing to do the right thing or hurting someone's feelings, and learn to think rationally about it.

Until now you've worked generally in regard to your guilt-related theme, the IBs that account for your guilt and developing your alternative RBs. However, to apply your general RBs in dealing with breaching your moral code or hurting someone's feelings, you must remember that since you make yourself guilty about specific events (actual or imagined), you should deal with these by rehearsing specific variants of your RBs.

The best way to do this is in specific situations with the people involved when you breached your moral code or whose feelings you hurt, but you may benefit by first using imagery as follows:

- Imagine a specific situation in which you felt guilty or may feel guilty about breaching your moral code or hurting someone's feelings; focus on what you felt most guilty about (i.e. your 'A').
- Focusing on 'A' while rehearsing a specific and relevant RB, try to make yourself feel remorseful but not guilty.
- Imagine yourself acting in ways consistent with your RB, e.g. apologize, make amends and engage the other person in a productive dialogue.
- Recognize that some of your post-belief thinking may be distorted. Respond without getting bogged down doing so. Accept the presence of any remaining distorted thoughts without engaging with them.
- Repeat these steps until you feel ready to put this sequence into practice in your life.

Apologize, make amends, talk things through

Having dealt with your guilt-related situation in imagery, you're ready to do so in reality, perhaps by apologizing to others for your behaviour and/or making amends. Whatever action is needed, first get into a rational frame of mind. When feeling remorseful but not guilty, engage others in a productive dialogue about the situation, if they're willing to do so, to achieve mutual understanding and reconciliation.

Capitalize on what you have learned and generalize your learning

When you've faced the situation in which you felt guilt and dealt with it as best you could, reflect on what you did and what you learned. In particular, if you were able to face the situation, rehearse your RBs and take constructive action, then ask yourself how you can capitalize on what you achieved and generalize your learning to similar situations.

Deal with any problems facing guilt-related situations

If you experienced problems facing what you were guilty about, answer the following:

- Did I face the situation? If not, why not?
- Did I rehearse my RBs before, during or after facing the situation? If not, why not?
- Did I execute my plan to face the situation? If not, why not?
- Did I engage with post-belief distorted thinking? If so, why?

Reflect on your experience and put into practice what you have learned the next time you face a situation in which you consider you have done the wrong thing, failed to do the right thing or hurt someone's feelings.

Become less guilt-prone

If you're particularly guilt-prone (i.e. experience guilt in a variety of different situations and limit your life to avoid feeling guilty), do the following.

Accept yourself unconditionally for being guilt-prone

If guilt-prone for whatever reason, you have an important choice to make at the outset: you can accept yourself unconditionally as a fallible human being, prone to experiencing guilt, or you can depreciate yourself for this proneness. Before making your choice, remember that unconditional self-acceptance doesn't mean you need to resign yourself to a lifetime of guilt-proneness. It means you're a fallible human being whether or not you're guilt-prone. It doesn't indicate that you cannot work to become less guilt-prone. Indeed, it helps you do this. If you depreciate yourself for being guilt-prone, you not only have emotional disturbance stemming from guilt-proneness, you're disturbing yourself about this disturbance: you have two disturbances for the price of one. So accepting yourself unconditionally for being guilt-prone not only spares you this secondary disturbance but helps you focus on your proneness with the purpose of helping you become less prone.

My advice then is: choose to accept yourself unconditionally for being guilt-prone.

Deal with emotional problems about guilt

In the same way as you may disturb yourself about being guilt-prone, you may also disturb yourself about specific instances of guilt by making yourself:

- anxious about the prospect of experiencing guilt;
- depressed about feeling guilt;
- ashamed about feeling guilt; or
- unhealthily angry with yourself for making yourself feel guilt.

See the chapters on anxiety, depression, shame and unhealthy anger for help if you tend to disturb yourself about feeling guilty.

Why you feel guilty much of the time and how to deal with this

If you're particularly guilt-prone you'll think you often do the wrong thing, fail to do the right thing or hurt others' feelings. This is because you hold a 'chronic guilt-based general IB': 'Whenever I'm involved, I must make sure nothing bad happens or others' feelings aren't hurt. If I don't and bad things happen and others are upset, it's all my fault and I'm a bad person.'

You then take this belief to relevant situations and, even where your involvement is minimal, you think you're at fault if there's a bad outcome. As a result you constantly think you're responsible for any negative outcomes and end up blaming yourself.

How to deal with chronic guilt

To deal with this chronic sense of guilt, you should develop and apply an alternative general RB to protect you from such guilt: 'Whenever I'm involved, I want to make sure nothing bad happens or that others' feelings aren't hurt, but I don't *have* to succeed in doing so. If I don't and bad things happen and others are upset, I'll take the appropriate responsibility, assign appropriate responsibility to others and consider the impact of situational factors. I'll accept myself for failing to adhere to my code and for any hurt I inadvertently cause.'

Such a belief will lead you to think you've breached your moral code or hurt someone's feelings only when there is clear evidence for making such an inference. When there is, you'll feel remorse rather than guilt, because you'll be processing this with a specific RB.

How to examine the accuracy of your guilt-related inference if necessary

If you're still unsure whether you've breached your moral code or hurt someone's feelings, answer one or more of the following questions:

- How valid is my inference that I breached my moral code (for example)?
- Would an objective jury agree that I breached my moral code? If not, what would their verdict be?
- Is my inference that I breached my moral code realistic? If not, what is a more realistic inference?
- If I asked someone I could trust to give me an objective opinion about my inference that I breached my moral code, what would that person say to me and why? What inference would he or she encourage me to make instead?
- If a friend told me she had made the same inference about breaching her moral code in the same situation, what would I say to her about the validity of her inference and why? What inference would I encourage her to make instead?

Understand the thinking consequences of your IBs

When you hold a set of IBs about breaching your moral code or hurting others' feelings, then, as discussed, a consequence is that your subsequent thinking is highly distorted and skewed to the negative.

If you don't understand how your mind works in this respect, you'll get caught up in your compelling distorted thoughts, regard them as representing reality and strive to protect yourself from what you regard as real negative events, rather than seeing them as highly distorted thinking consequences of IBs you've created.

However, if you do understand this phenomenon and act on this understanding, you'll trace such thinking back to the IBs that spawned it and will do one of two things (or both):

- question these IBs;
- acknowledge the existence of such distorted thinking and go about your business while neither engaging with it nor trying to eliminate it; you'll maintain this understanding no matter how compelling your distorted thoughts are.

Other ways of becoming less guilt-prone
Practise healthy self-care

People with guilt problems tend to put others first because they think that putting themselves first is selfish, and lack a philosophy of healthy self-care comprising the following principles:

- Healthy self-care is flexible. It involves you putting yourself first most of the time and putting the interests of others you care about a close second; it sometimes involves you putting the interests of others first.
- Putting yourself first is not selfish since you also care about others.
- You're not a bad person if you put yourself first.
- If you don't look after yourself, nobody else will do the job for you.

To become less guilt-prone you should act on those principles listed above.

Give up hidden conceit

Guilt often involves conceit. This happens when you think you're a bad person for doing something wrong but you don't think of another person in that way for doing the same thing. Why is this conceit? Because you're saying, in effect, that the other person is a fallible human being, allowed to do the wrong thing, while you're a bad person and absolutely shouldn't have done it, and you expect higher moral standards from yourself than you do from others. Thus, another way of becoming less guilt-prone is to expect yourself to be as human as others.

Realize that you don't hurt others' feelings

If you're guilt-prone, you often think you hurt others' feelings and that you're bad for doing so. To deal with your guilt about hurting others, I've shown that you need to assume temporarily that you do so and then think rationally about this. When you've done this, you need to understand that you don't hurt others' feelings – they hurt themselves about your treatment of them. If you accept this principle, you can think more clearly about your behaviour towards these others without assuming that, if they're hurt, it's your fault. Of course, adopting this principle doesn't give you carte blanche to treat others badly, assuming that they are responsible for their own feelings. It means that you're responsible for how you act towards others, and if your behaviour towards others is reasonable and they feel hurt about it, then they need to take responsibility for their own feelings.

Summary

You can make yourself less guilt-prone by:

- accepting yourself unconditionally for being guilt-prone;
- dealing effectively with your emotional problems about guilt;
- developing a healthy attitude towards your involvement in events when things go wrong so you can make realistic inferences at 'A' about the extent to which you breached your moral code or hurt others' feelings;
- understanding that when you hold IBs about breaching your moral code or hurting others' feelings, you exaggerate the nature of your behaviour and its consequences; however, you will not engage with such thinking but trace it back to the IBs that spawned it, which you'll challenge; you'll then let any remnants of such thinking be, again without engaging with it or trying to eliminate it;
- implementing the philosophy of healthy self-care;
- expecting the same moral standards from yourself as you do from others;
- treating others well and allowing them to take responsibility for their own hurt feelings.

In the next chapter, I deal with the deadly emotion known as shame.

5

Dealing with shame

Shame is a deadly emotion that, like guilt, stops you from taking risks and leads you to live a restricted life where you hide important aspects of yourself from others. This chapter outlines the RECBT view of shame and its healthy alternative, disappointment, before showing you what you need to do to deal effectively with this deadly emotion.

Understanding shame

This section discusses the RECBT view of what happens when you make yourself ashamed and how to deal effectively with this deadly emotion, using RECBT's 'ABC' model where 'A' stands for 'adversity', 'B' for beliefs and 'C' for the consequences of these beliefs. However, I will use the order 'CAB' since it's best to start with features of shame at 'C'.

'C'

Chapter 1 explained that there are three main features of any emotional problem: feeling, behavioural and thinking. If you're shame-prone you often feel anxious in case something happens about which you experience shame. When you actually experience shame, your feelings are closely linked to your wish to disappear or become invisible. This is also reflected in your behaviour.

Behaviour associated with shame

When feeling shame, you tend to act in several ways, outlined in Table 5.1. Most of these behaviours are designed to remove you from public view, and/or protect your threatened self-esteem.

Thinking associated with shame

When feeling shame, you tend to think in ways that exaggerate the nature and consequences of what you feel ashamed about in the first place (see Table 5.1 for a full list of thinking that accompanies shame).

Table 5.1 Shame vs disappointment

Adversity	• Something highly negative has been revealed about you (or about a group with whom you identify) by yourself or by others. • You have acted in a way that falls very short of your ideal. • Others look down on or shun you (or a group with whom you identify) or you think that they do.	
Belief	IRRATIONAL	RATIONAL
Emotion	Shame	Disappointment
Behaviour	• You remove yourself from the 'gaze' of others. • You isolate yourself from others. • You save face by attacking other(s) who have 'shamed' you. • You defend your threatened self-esteem in self-defeating ways. • You ignore attempts by others to restore social equilibrium.	• You continue to participate actively in social interaction. • You respond positively to attempts of others to restore social equilibrium.
Subsequent thinking	• You overestimate the negativity of the information revealed. • You overestimate the likelihood that the judging group will notice or be interested in the information. • You overestimate the degree of disapproval you (or your reference group) will receive. • You overestimate how long any disapproval will last.	• You see the information revealed in a compassionate self-accepting context. • You are realistic about the likelihood that the judging group will notice or be interested in the information revealed. • You are realistic about the degree of disapproval you (or your reference group) will receive. • You are realistic about how long any disapproval will last.

'A'

Chapter 1 explained that 'A' stands for adversity: what you're most disturbed about with respect to your personal domain. When feeling shame, the inferences you make (what you feel ashamed about) have to do with the social-behavioural realm of your personal domain and how you and others with whom you're closely identified are viewed within this realm. Thus, you think that:

• something highly negative has been revealed about you (or about a group with whom you identify) by yourself or by others;

- you've acted in a way that falls very short of your ideal;
- others look down on or shun you (or a group with whom you identify) or you think they do.

As with all deadly emotions, when you feel shame, you think your inferences are facts.

'B'

As Chapter 1 explained, beliefs are at the heart of the RECBT model of the emotions. When you make one or more of the three shame-related inferences listed, these inferences on their own don't explain your shame, since, as I'll show, it's possible and desirable for you to feel disappointment when (1) something highly negative has been revealed about you (or a group with whom you identify) by yourself or others; (2) you've acted in a way that falls very short of your ideal; and/or (3) you think others look down on or shun you (or a group with whom you identify). Chapter 1 indicated that you can hold a set of IBs or RBs about adversity.

IBs about shame-related inferences

The RECBT model of shame is that you feel ashamed that (1) something highly negative has been revealed about you (or a group with whom you identify) by yourself or others; (2) you've acted in a way that falls very short of your ideal; and/or (3) you think that others look down on or shun you (or a group with whom you identify) when you hold IBs about these shame-related inferences. These beliefs are rigid and extreme in that you depreciate yourself as defective, diminished or disgusting.

Understanding disappointment

As Chapter 1 explained, when you face a negative event it is healthy for you to experience a negative emotion that helps you deal effectively with the negative event you face. This section discusses the RECBT view of disappointment as the healthy alternative to shame, again using the 'CABDE' order of the 'ABCDE' framework.

'C'

As explained above, there are three main features of shame: feeling, behavioural and thinking. The same is true when you're feeling disappointment but not shame. Thus, you may feel symptoms related to concern in anticipation of something happening about which you feel disappointment. When you actually experience disappointment, your feelings are closely linked to your wish to stay in the situation. This is also reflected in your behaviour. These feelings will encourage you to think clearly about your shame-related inference and motivate you to take constructive action.

Behaviour associated with disappointment

When feeling disappointed but not ashamed, you're motivated to face what you feel disappointment about and deal with it. Table 5.1 outlines the major ways you feel like acting when disappointed.

Thinking associated with disappointment

When feeling disappointed but not ashamed, you tend to think in ways designed to help you face and deal effectively with what you feel disappointed about. Such thinking tends to be realistic and balanced (see Table 5.1).

'A'

When feeling disappointed but not ashamed, the themes about which you feel disappointed are the same as those about which you feel shame, namely: (1) something highly negative has been revealed about you (or a group with whom you identify) by yourself or others; (2) you've acted in a way that falls very short of your ideal; and/or (3) you think others look down on or shun you (or a group with whom you identify) – see Table 5.1.

'B'

When you feel disappointed but not ashamed, (1) that something highly negative has been revealed about you (or a group with whom you identify) by yourself or others, (2) that you've acted in a way that falls very short of your ideal; and/or (3) you think that others look down on or shun you (or a group with whom you identify), you do so because the beliefs that you hold about these inferences are rational.

RBs about shame-related inferences

The RECBT model of disappointment is that you feel disappointed but not ashamed about: (1) something highly negative that has been revealed about you (or a group with whom you identify) by yourself or by others; (2) your acting in a way that falls very short of your ideal; and/or (3) your thinking that others look down on or shun you (or a group with whom you identify), when you hold RBs about these inferences. These beliefs are flexible and non-extreme in that you accept yourself as fallible.

How to deal with shame

Since you make yourself ashamed about (1) something highly negative being revealed about you (or a group with whom you identify) by yourself or by others, (2) having acted in a way that falls very short of your ideal; and/or (3) thinking that others look down on or shun you (or a group with whom you identify), your goal is to make yourself feel disappointed but not ashamed about these inferences. This is why I'll be encouraging you to assume temporarily that your shame-related inferences at 'A' are correct. Once you're disappointed rather than ashamed, you'll be in a sufficiently rational frame of mind to examine your shame-related inferences. If you're ashamed about them you will not be objective enough while examining your inferences. Later, I will also explain why you're prone to your shame-related thinking in ambiguous situations and will help you to become less prone.

Ensure that you're feeling shame and it's a problem for you

Before you do anything to try to change your feelings of shame, ensure that you're feeling shame and that you see that shame is a problem for you. Otherwise, you'll resist your own efforts to help yourself.

Are you feeling shame?

People use the term 'shame' loosely; if you say you feel ashamed, you may or may not be experiencing the deadly version of this emotion. Determine whether you're experiencing the deadly version of shame by consulting the behavioural and thinking consequences of both IBs and RBs about: (1) something highly negative that has been revealed about you (or a group with whom you identify) by yourself or others; (2) your having acted in a way that falls very short of your ideal; and/or (3) you think that others look down on or shun you (or a group with whom you identify). The more your behaviour and thinking match those listed in Table 5.1 as consequences of IBs, the more likely you are (or were) feeling shame rather than disappointment. Conversely, the more your behaviour and thinking match those listed as consequences of RBs, the more likely you are (or were) feeling disappointment rather than shame.

Is shame a problem for you?

Assuming you've determined that you experienced shame rather than disappointment, now determine whether or not you consider your shame is a problem you want to change. Just because your experience matches those listed in Table 5.1 as shame, this doesn't mean you'll inevitably see it's a problem for you.

If you are uncertain whether shame is a problem for you, answer the following:

- Does my shame help me to deal effectively with:
  - something highly negative being revealed about me (or a group with whom I identify) by myself or others?
  - my acting in a way that falls very short of my ideal?

- when I think others look down on or shun me (or a group with whom I identify)?
- Does my shame help me to compassionately contextualize my behaviour or that of others with whom I closely identify?

If you've answered 'yes' to either or both questions, you may be reluctant to target your shame for change. I suggest you read the following section with an open mind and then answer two different questions.

Commit to disappointment as a productive alternative to shame

In any self-change venture, you need clear alternatives to problems you wish to change. Otherwise you'll be in a 'change vacuum', where you know what you don't want to feel but don't know what it would be healthy for you to feel instead. RECBT argues that when you face (or think you are facing) a situation where (1) something highly negative has been revealed about you (or a group with whom you identify) by yourself or by others, and/or (2) you've acted in a way that falls very short of your ideal; and/or (3) others look down on or shun you (or a group with whom you identify), the healthy alternative to feeling shame is disappointment. Table 5.1 lists the behavioural and thinking consequences of RBs about the above situations which may trigger you to feel disappointment. If you see that these consequences help you to deal effectively with the inferences I have listed, then you're ready to commit yourself to feeling disappointed rather than ashamed about these inferences.

For those ambivalent about targeting shame as a problem to change in the previous section, answer the following questions while consulting the relevant sections of Table 5.1:

- Does shame or disappointment help me deal effectively with:
  - something highly negative being revealed about me (or a group with whom I identify) by myself or by others?
  - my acting in a way that falls very short of my ideal?
  - when I think that others look down on or shun me (or a group with whom I identify)?
- Does shame or disappointment help me compassionately contextualize my behaviour or that of others with whom I closely identify?

Hopefully, if you were ambivalent about targeting your shame for change, you're now ready to do so and to work towards feeling disappointment rather than shame about your shame-related inferences.

Identify what you are most ashamed about at 'A'

If you have a problem with shame, you're likely to experience this deadly emotion in situations where you infer that:

- something highly negative has been revealed about you (or about a group with whom you identify) by yourself or others;
- you've acted in a way that falls very short of your ideal;
- others look down on or shun you (or a group with whom you identify).

To identify your shame-related inference, ask yourself such questions as:

- What did I feel most ashamed about in the situation I was in?
- When I felt shame:
  - what negative thing about me (or others with whom I identify) was revealed?
  - in what way did I think I fell very short of my ideal?
  - what did I think others thought about me (or others with whom I identify)?

Use the 'magic question' technique

If you still cannot identify your shame-related inference, use the 'magic question' technique:

- Focus on the situation in which you felt ashamed.
- Without changing the situation, ask yourself: 'What one thing would eliminate or significantly reduce my shame?'
- The opposite is what you're most ashamed about.

Here's how Peter used this technique:

- I felt ashamed when I got a lower second degree.
- If I didn't think I had significantly underperformed, I wouldn't have felt ashamed.
- I felt most ashamed about significantly underperforming on my degree.

Identify the IBs underpinning your shame and the rational alternatives underpinning disappointment

The RECBT model argues that shame-related inferences don't make you feel ashamed. Rather, you make yourself feel ashamed by holding IBs (at 'B') about these inferences and if you hold RBs (also at 'B') about them instead, then you'll feel disappointment but not shame.

Consequently, you should identify your IBs about your shame-related inferences at 'A' and the rational alternatives to these IBs. I recommend the latter so you can derive hope that you can see there's an alternative to the main determining factor of your shame.

In identifying your IBs, specify your rigid belief and extreme self-depreciation belief, and in identifying your alternative RBs, specify your flexible belief and non-extreme unconditional self-acceptance belief.

Acknowledge the 'B–C' connection

Before proceeding to question these beliefs, it is useful for you to acknowledge the connection between your IBs (at 'B') and your shame (at 'C') and between your RBs (also at 'B') and your feelings of disappointment (at 'E') that you're aiming to experience in response to (1) something highly negative having been revealed about you (or about a group with whom you identify) by yourself or by others; (2) your acting in a way that falls very short of your ideal; and/or (3) when you think others have looked down on or shunned you (or a group with whom you identify).

Question your beliefs

You're now ready to question your beliefs to see clearly that your IBs are irrational (i.e. false, illogical and largely unhelpful) and that your alternative RBs are rational (i.e. true, logical and largely helpful). To enable you to get the most out of this process:

- Begin by questioning your rigid belief and flexible belief together. Ask yourself:
  - Which of these beliefs is true? Which is false?
  - Which of these beliefs is logical? Which is illogical?
  - Which of these beliefs is largely helpful? Which is largely unhelpful?

  Provide reasons for your answers. See Appendix 2 for suggestions concerning arguments on this issue. You'll need to tailor your arguments to the content of your beliefs.
- Take your self-depreciation belief and unconditional self-acceptance belief and question them by asking the same three questions as above. Again provide reasons for your answers. See Appendix 3 for suggestions concerning arguments on this issue, which have to be tailored to the content of your beliefs.

Having completed this process you should understand why your IBs are irrational and why the rational alternatives to these beliefs are rational, and will be in a position to commit yourself to act and think in ways consistent with your RBs to enable you to deal effectively when a situation triggers in you feelings of shame.

Adopt a healthy orientation towards your high standards

Having committed yourself to strengthening your conviction in your RBs, you should develop a healthy orientation towards your high standards as follows:

- Recognize that there's nothing intrinsically wrong with having high standards.
- View these standards as signposts to aim for rather than yardsticks you must achieve. As such, your high standards are similar to self-actualization in that you can never achieve them once and for all. Rather, you can work steadily to achieve them.
- Accept that when you fail to live up to your high standards, the best way of dealing with this situation is to learn from it and apply your learning on future occasions, having first accepted yourself unconditionally for your failure.

Face your shame-related theme in imagery

Assuming you've committed to act on your RBs (flexible belief and unconditional self-acceptance belief), you must face up to (1) something highly negative being revealed about you (or about a group with whom you identify) by yourself or by others; (2) your having acted in a way that falls very short of your ideal; and/or (3) when you think others look down on or shun you (or a group with whom you identify) and learn to think rationally about it.

Until now you've worked generally in regard to your shame-related theme, the IBs that account for your shame and developing your alternative RBs. However, to apply your RBs when a situation triggers feelings of shame as described above, you must remember that since you make yourself ashamed about specific events (actual or imagined), you should deal with these by rehearsing specific variants of your RBs.

The best way to do this is in specific situations with the people involved when your feelings of shame are triggered, as described above, but you may benefit by first using imagery as follows:

- Imagine a specific situation in which you felt ashamed or may feel ashamed when
  - something highly negative has been revealed about you (or about a group with whom you identify) by yourself or by others;
  - you have acted in a way that falls very short of your ideal; and/or
  - you think others look down on or shun you (or a group with whom you identify).
  Focus on what you felt most ashamed about (i.e. your 'A') while rehearsing a specific and relevant RB. Try to make yourself feel disappointed but not ashamed.
- Imagine yourself acting in ways consistent with your RB, e.g. holding your head up high and dealing with relevant issues with relevant people rather than hiding away from them.
- Recognize that some of your post-belief thinking may be distorted. Respond without getting bogged down doing so. Accept the presence

of any remaining distorted thoughts without engaging with them.
- Repeat these steps until you feel ready to put this sequence into practice in your life.

Face situations and people with your head held high

Having learned the lessons from previous shame-based episodes, you're ready to return to the social milieu: hold your head up as you do so.

- Choose a specific situation that reminds you of your humiliation and about which you would ordinarily feel ashamed.
- Rehearse a specific version of your general RBs before entering the situation so you're prepared to face the music in a rational frame of mind.
- Develop a shortened version of this RB in your mind as you enter the situation (e.g. 'I'm still fallible even though I feel humiliated'), accepting that you're likely to be uncomfortable doing so. React to any consequences with a rational frame of mind if possible.
- Recognize that even though you've got yourself into a rational frame of mind, some of your thinking may be distorted/unrealistic, some may be realistic/balanced. Accept the presence of the former and don't engage with it; engage with the latter as much as possible.

Capitalize on what you have learned and generalize your learning

When you've faced the situation in which you felt shame and dealt with it as best you could, reflect on what you did and what you have learned. In particular, if you were able to face the situation, rehearse your RBs and take constructive action, then ask yourself how you can capitalize on what you achieved and generalize your learning to similar situations.

Deal with any problems facing shame-related situations

If you experienced problems facing what you were ashamed about, answer the following:

- Did I face the situation? If not, why not?
- Did I rehearse my RBs before, during or after facing the situation? If not, why not?
- Did I execute my plan to face the situation? If not, why not?
- Did I engage with post-belief distorted thinking? If so, why?

Reflect on your experience and put into practice what you have learned next time you face a situation where (1) something highly negative has been revealed about you (or about a group with whom you identify) by yourself or by others; (2) you've acted in a way that falls very short of your ideal; and/or (3) you think others look down on or shun you (or a group with whom you identify).

Become less shame-prone

If you're particularly shame-prone (i.e. experience shame in a variety of different situations and limit your life to avoid feeling shame), do the following.

Accept yourself unconditionally for being shame-prone

If shame-prone for whatever reason, you have an important choice to make at the outset: you can accept yourself unconditionally as a fallible human being, prone to experiencing shame, or you can depreciate yourself for this proneness. Before you make your choice, remember that unconditional self-acceptance doesn't mean you need to resign yourself to a lifetime of shame-proneness. It means you're a fallible human being whether or not you're shame-prone. It doesn't indicate that you cannot work to become less shame-prone. Indeed, it helps you do this. If you depreciate yourself for being shame-prone, you not only have emotional disturbance stemming from shame-proneness, you're disturbing yourself about this disturbance: you have two disturbances for the price of one. So accepting yourself unconditionally for being shame-prone not only spares you this secondary disturbance but helps you focus on your proneness with the purpose of helping you become less prone.

My advice then is: choose to accept yourself unconditionally for being shame-prone.

Deal with emotional problems about shame

In the same way that you may disturb yourself about being shame-prone, you may also disturb yourself about specific instances of shame by making yourself:

• anxious about the prospect of experiencing shame;
• depressed about feeling shame;
• ashamed about feeling shame; or
• unhealthily angry with yourself for making yourself feel shame.

See the chapters on anxiety, depression and unhealthy anger for help if you tend to disturb yourself about feeling shame.

Deal with meta-shame

When you feel ashamed about experiencing shame, you see your original shame as a weakness and hold a set of IBs about it (e.g. 'I mustn't have this weakness and because I do, this proves I'm a weak, defective person'). Question these beliefs and develop conviction in alternative RBs (e.g. 'I'd prefer not to feel shame as it's a weakness, but I'm not immune from this feeling, nor do I have to be immune. I'm not a weak, defective person for having this weakness. I'm a fallible, complex, unrateable person who has strengths and weaknesses'). Owning up to your meta-shame and accepting yourself unconditionally for experiencing it will help you face up to and address your original shame in the same way.

Why you're prone to shame and how to deal with this

If you're particularly prone to shame you'll think that (1) you (or people with whom you closely identify) often reveal something highly negative about you; (2) you often act in a way that falls very short of your ideal; and/or (3) others often look down on or shun you (or those with whom you closely identify). This is because you hold a 'chronic shame-based general IB': 'I must ensure that I and people with whom I'm closely connected must always achieve the highest of standards and be socially approved; if not, it proves we're defective, disgusting or diminished.'

You then take this belief to situations where it's possible you and others will fall short or be socially disapproved, and you attempt to protect all involved from the predicted negative outcomes by getting all to maintain standards or withdraw so that social approval is maintained. However, in doing so, you're keeping alive the three inferences of shame. For you're saying to yourself that if you didn't take the appropriate steps:

- something highly negative would be revealed about you (or a group with whom you identify) by yourself or by others;
- you'd act in a way that falls very short of your ideal; and
- others would look down on or shun you (or a group with whom you identify).

How to deal with chronic shame

To deal with this chronic sense of shame, you should develop and apply an alternative general RB to protect you from such shame: 'I'd like to ensure that I and people with whom I'm closely connected always achieve the highest standards and are socially approved, but I don't have to do so. If I didn't it would be unfortunate, but it would prove we're not defective, disgusting or diminished. Rather, it would prove we're fallible human beings and that doesn't change whether or not we're humiliated and disapproved of.'

Such a belief will lead you to think that the following occurred only when there is clear evidence for making such an inference:

- something highly negative has been revealed about you (or about a group with whom you identify) by yourself or by others;
- you've acted in a way that falls very short of your ideal; and
- others look down on or shun you (or a group with whom you identify) or you think that they do.

When there's such evidence you'll feel disappointment rather than shame because you'll be processing this with a specific RB.

How to examine the accuracy of your shame-related inference if necessary

If you're still unsure that (1) something highly negative has been revealed about you (or about a group with whom you identify) by yourself or by others; (2) you've acted in a way that falls very short of your ideal; and (3) others look down on or shun you (or a group with whom you identify), answer one or more of the following questions:

- How valid is my inference that I've fallen very short of my ideal (for example)?
- Would an objective jury agree that I've fallen very short of my ideal? If not, what would their verdict be?
- Is my inference that I've fallen very short of my ideal realistic? If not, what is a more realistic inference?
- If I asked someone I could trust to give me an objective opinion about my inference that I've fallen very short of my ideal, what would that person say to me and why? What inference would he or she encourage me to make instead?
- If a friend told me he had made the same inference about falling very short of his ideal in the same situation, what would I say to him about the validity of his inference and why? What inference would I encourage him to make instead?

Understand the thinking consequences of your IBs

When you hold a set of IBs about one or more shame-based inferences then, as discussed, a consequence is that your subsequent thinking is highly distorted and skewed to the negative.

If you don't understand how your mind works in this respect, you'll get caught up in your compelling distorted thoughts and will regard them as representing reality, and will strive to protect yourself from what you regard as real negative events rather than seeing them as highly distorted thinking consequences of IBs you've created.

However, if you do understand this phenomenon and act on this understanding, you'll trace such thinking back to the IBs that spawned it and you will do one of two things (or both):

- question these IBs;
- acknowledge the existence of such distorted thinking and go about your business while neither engaging with it nor trying to eliminate it; you'll maintain this understanding no matter how compelling your distorted thoughts are.

See that you can hold an individual sense of 'I' in the face of a socially defined 'I'

In shame, you tend to define yourself as others define you or as you think they define you. If this is the case then you need to develop an individual sense of 'I' in the face of an actual or inferred negative socially defined 'I'. For example, if others define you as defective for displaying a weakness (or you think they do), you need to define yourself differently (e.g. 'I'm not defective for displaying this weakness. I'm fallible'). Developing a rational individually defined 'I' is very important as you strive to become less shame-prone.

Summary

You can make yourself less shame-prone by:

- accepting yourself unconditionally for being shame-prone;
- dealing effectively with your emotional problems about shame;
- developing RBs about yourself failing to reach ideal standards which will enable you to make realistic inferences at 'A' about your behaviour, the behaviour of others with whom you closely identify and the attitude of observing others in given situations;
- understanding that when you hold IBs about your shame-based inferences, you'll exaggerate the nature of your behaviour and its consequences as well as the way others evaluate you. However, you will not engage with such thinking but trace it back to the IBs that spawned it, which you will challenge; you'll then let any remnants of such thinking be, again without engaging with it or trying to eliminate it;
- developing and implementing a rational individual sense of 'I'.

In the next chapter, I deal with the deadly emotion known as hurt.

6

Dealing with hurt

This chapter outlines the RECBT view of hurt and its healthy alternative, sorrow, before showing you what you need to do to deal effectively with this deadly emotion.

Understanding hurt

This chapter discusses the RECBT view of what happens when you make yourself hurt and how to deal effectively with this deadly emotion, using RECBT's 'ABC' model where 'A' stands for 'adversity', 'B' for beliefs and 'C' for the consequences of these beliefs. However, I will use the order 'CAB' since it's best to start with features of hurt at 'C'.

'C'

Chapter 1 explained that there are three main features of any emotional problem: feeling, behavioural and thinking. You're likely to feel hurt in several ways. Common experiences include depression, self-pity, unhealthy anger and a non-specific emotional pain. These feelings tend to interfere with your thinking clearly about what you feel hurt about and to impede constructive action.

Behaviour associated with hurt

When feeling hurt, you tend to act in certain ways, outlined in Table 6.1.

Thinking associated with hurt

When feeling hurt, you tend to think in ways that exaggerate what you originally felt hurt about and also what you see as its likely consequences (see Table 6.1 for a full list of thinking that accompanies hurt).

'A'

Chapter 1 explained that 'A' stands for adversity: what you're most disturbed about with respect to your personal domain. When feeling hurt, you make one or more of the following inferences:

- others treat you badly (and you think you don't deserve such treatment);

Table 6.1 Hurt vs sorrow

Adversity	• Others treat you badly (and you think you do not deserve such treatment).	
	• You think that the other person has devalued your relationship (i.e. someone indicates that his or her relationship with you is less important to him or her than the relationship is to you).	
Belief	**IRRATIONAL**	**RATIONAL**
Emotion	**Hurt**	**Sorrow**
Behaviour	• You stop communicating with the other person. • You sulk and make it obvious that you feel hurt without disclosing details of the matter. • You indirectly criticize or punish the other person for his or her offence.	• You communicate your feelings to the other person directly. • You request that the other person acts in a fairer manner towards you.
Subsequent thinking	• You overestimate the unfairness of the other person's behaviour. • You think that the other person does not care for you or is indifferent to you. • You see yourself as alone, uncared for or misunderstood. • You tend to think of past 'hurts'.	• You are realistic about the degree of unfairness in the other person's behaviour. • You think that the other person has acted badly rather than that he or she has demonstrated a lack of caring or indifference. • You see yourself as being in a poor situation, but still connected to, cared for by and understood by others not directly involved in the situation. • If you think of past hurts you do so with less frequency and less intensity than when you feel hurt. • You are open to the idea of making the first move towards the other person.

- you think the other person has devalued your relationship (i.e. someone indicates that his or her relationship with you is less important to him or her than the relationship is to you).

Such hurt-related inferences may occur in either the ego realm or the non-ego realm of your personal domain.

'B'

As Chapter 1 explained, beliefs are at the heart of the RECBT model of the emotions. Undeserved bad treatment from others and/or relationship devaluation, on their own, do not explain your hurt since, as I'll show, it's possible and desirable to feel sorrowful about these inferences. As Chapter 1 indicated, you can hold a set of IBs or RBs about adversity.

IBs about undeserved bad treatment and/or relationship devaluation

The RECBT model of hurt is that you feel hurt about undeserved bad treatment from others and/or relationship devaluation when you hold IBs about them. These beliefs are rigid and extreme. Please note:

- rigid beliefs are common to both ego hurt and non-ego hurt;
- self-depreciation beliefs are the main extreme beliefs in ego hurt;
- awfulizing beliefs or discomfort intolerance beliefs are the main extreme beliefs in non-ego hurt; in this form of hurt, self-pity is a strong element.

Understanding sorrow

As Chapter 1 explained, when you face a negative event it's healthy to experience a negative emotion that helps you deal effectively with the negative event you face. This section discusses the RECBT view of sorrow as the healthy alternative to hurt, again using the 'CABDE' order of the 'ABCDE' framework.

'C'

As explained above, there are three main features of hurt: feeling, behavioural and thinking. The same is true when you're sorrowful but not hurt. When sorrowful, you may have feelings such as sadness and healthy anger which will encourage you to think clearly about the way you've been treated and the way the other person sees your relationship and motivates you to take constructive action.

Behaviour associated with sorrow

When feeling sorrowful but not hurt, you're motivated to face the person who has treated you badly or devalued your relationship and discuss the issue with him or her. Table 6.1 outlines the major ways you act or feel like acting when you feel sorrowful.

Thinking associated with sorrow

When you feel sorrowful but not hurt, you tend to think in ways designed to help you face and deal effectively with the situation threat (see Table 6.1).

'A'

When you feel sorrow but not hurt, what you feel sorrowful about is the same as you feel hurt about, i.e. undeserved bad treatment and/or relationship devaluation (see Table 6.1).

'B'

When you feel sorrow but not hurt about undeserved bad treatment and/or relationship devaluation, you do so because the beliefs you hold about these inferences are rational.

RBs about undeserved bad treatment and/or relationship devaluation

The RECBT model of sorrow is to feel sorrow but not hurt about undeserved bad treatment and/or relationship devaluation when you hold RBs about these inferences. These beliefs are flexible and non-extreme. Please note:

- flexible beliefs are common to both ego sorrow and non-ego sorrow;
- unconditional self-acceptance beliefs are the main non-extreme beliefs in ego sorrow;
- non-awfulizing beliefs or discomfort tolerance beliefs are the main non-extreme beliefs in non-ego sorrow.

How to deal with hurt

Since you make yourself hurt about undeserved bad treatment and/or relationship devaluation, your goal is to make yourself sorrowful, concerned, but not hurt about these inferences. That's why I'll encourage you to assume temporarily that your inferences of undeserved bad treatment or relationship devaluation at 'A' are correct. Once you're sorrowful rather than hurt, you'll be in a sufficiently rational frame of mind to examine your hurt-related inferences. If you're hurt about these inferences, you won't be objective enough while examining them. Later, I'll explain why you're prone to inferring the existence of undeserved bad treatment and/or relationship devaluation in ambiguous situations and will help you become less prone.

Ensure that you're feeling hurt and it's a problem for you

Before doing anything to try to change hurt feelings, ensure that you're feeling hurt and that you see hurt is a problem for you. Otherwise, you'll resist your own efforts to help yourself.

Do you feel hurt?

People use the term 'hurt' loosely; if you say you feel hurt, you may or may not be experiencing the deadly version of this emotion. Determine whether you're experiencing the deadly version by consulting the behavioural and thinking consequences of both IBs and RBs about undeserved bad treatment and relationship devaluation. The more your behaviour and thinking match those listed in Table 6.1 as consequences of IBs, the more likely you feel/felt hurt, rather than sorrowful. Conversely, the more your behaviour and thinking match those listed as consequences of RBs, the more likely you feel/felt sorrowful rather than hurt.

Is your hurt a problem for you?

Assuming you've determined that you experienced hurt rather than sorrow, now determine whether or not you consider your hurt a problem you want to change. Just because your experience matches those listed in Table 6.1 as hurt doesn't mean you'll inevitably see it as a problem for you.

If you're uncertain whether hurt is a problem for you, answer the following:

• Does my hurt help me deal effectively with the undeserved bad treatment I experienced or the other person devaluing our relationship?
• Does my hurt motivate me to engage the other person in a productive dialogue?

If you've answered 'yes' to either or both questions, you may be reluctant to target your hurt for change. Read the following section with an open mind and then answer two different questions.

Commit to sorrow as a productive alternative to hurt

In any self-change venture, you need clear alternatives to problems you wish to change. Otherwise you'll be in a 'change vacuum', where you know what you don't want to feel but don't know what it would be healthy for you to feel instead. RECBT argues that when you face (or think you're facing) undeserved bad treatment from someone close to you or when that person devalues his or her relationship with you, then the healthy alternative to feeling hurt about these inferences is to feel sorrowful about them. Table 6.1 lists the behavioural and thinking consequences of RBs about undeserved bad treatment and relationship devaluation associated with sorrow. If you see that these consequences help you deal effectively with such undeserved bad treatment and relationship devaluation, you're ready to commit yourself to feeling sorrow rather than hurt about these inferences.

For those ambivalent about targeting hurt as a problem to change in the previous section, answer the following questions while consulting the relevant sections of Table 6.1:

- Will hurt or sorrow help me deal more effectively with undeserved bad treatment and/or relationship devaluation?
- Which will help me more to engage the other person in a productive dialogue: hurt or sorrow?

Hopefully, if you were previously ambivalent about targeting your hurt for change, you're now ready to do so and to work towards feeling sorrow rather than hurt about undeserved bad treatment and/or relationship devaluation.

Identify what you're most hurt about at 'A'

If you have a problem with hurt, you're likely to experience this deadly emotion in situations where you infer that someone close to you has treated you badly and undeservedly and/or thinks less of your relationship than you do. For our purposes in this chapter, there are two realms of your personal domain:

- the ego realm, where you infer the presence of these two situations as impacting on your self-esteem;
- the non-ego realm, where you infer the presence of these two situations as impacting on your sense of comfort, broadly defined.

Such inferences can exist in both realms. To identify what you're hurt about, ask yourself:

- What was I most hurt about in the situation I was in?
- Did I think that the other person treated me badly in a way I didn't deserve? If so, what did he or she do?
- Did I consider the other person thought less of our relationship than I do? If so, what gave me that impression?

Use the 'magic question' technique

If you still cannot identify your hurt-related inference, use the 'magic question' technique:

- Focus on the situation in which you felt hurt.
- Without changing the situation, ask yourself: 'What one thing would have eliminated or significantly reduced my hurt feelings?'
- The opposite is what you were most hurt about.

Here's how Gina used this technique:

- I felt hurt when my friends went out together without asking me to go with them.
- If I'd known they weren't neglecting me, I wouldn't have felt hurt.
- I was most hurt about my friends neglecting me.

Identify the IBs underpinning your hurt and the rational alternatives underpinning sorrow

The RECBT model argues that undeserved bad treatment and/or relationship devaluation within your personal domain don't make you feel hurt. Rather, you make yourself hurt by holding IBs (at 'B') about these inferences, and if you hold RBs (also at 'B') about them instead, then you'll feel sorrow but not hurt.

Consequently, you should identify your IBs about the undeserved bad treatment you received or the relationship devaluation at 'A' and also the rational alternatives to these IBs. I recommend doing the latter so you can derive hope that you can see there's an alternative to the main determining factor of your hurt feelings.

In identifying your IBs and alternative RBs, determine whether your hurt is ego-related, impacting on your self-esteem, or non-ego-related, impacting on your sense of comfort, broadly defined, and not impacting on your self-esteem. Then do the following.

Ego hurt

If your hurt is ego-related, identify your rigid belief and your self-depreciation belief about undeserved bad treatment and/or relationship devaluation. Then identify their rational alternatives, i.e. your flexible belief and unconditional self-acceptance belief.

Non-ego hurt

If your hurt is non-ego-related, identify your rigid belief and either your awfulizing belief or your discomfort intolerance belief about undeserved bad treatment and/or relationship devaluation. These can also involve self-pity beliefs ('poor me'). Then identify their rational alternatives, i.e. your flexible belief and either your non-awfulizing belief or your discomfort tolerance belief.

Acknowledge the 'B–C' connection

Before proceeding to question these beliefs, acknowledge the connection between your IBs (at 'B') and your hurt (at 'C') and between your RBs (also at 'B') and your feelings of sorrow (at 'E') that you're aiming to experience in response to the undeserved bad treatment and/or relationship devaluation (at 'A').

Question your beliefs

You're now ready to question your beliefs to see clearly that your IBs are irrational (i.e. false, illogical and largely unhelpful) and that your alternative RBs are rational (i.e. true, logical and largely helpful). To enable you to get the most out of this process:

- Begin by questioning your rigid belief and flexible belief together. Ask yourself:
  - Which of these beliefs is true? Which is false?
  - Which of these beliefs is logical? Which is illogical?
  - Which of these beliefs is largely helpful? Which is largely unhelpful?

  Provide reasons for your answers. See Appendix 2 for suggestions concerning arguments on this issue. You'll need to tailor your arguments to the content of your beliefs.
- If your hurt is ego-based, take your self-depreciation belief and unconditional self-acceptance belief and question them by asking the same three questions as above. Again provide reasons for your answers. See Appendix 3 for suggestions concerning arguments on this issue, which have to be tailored to the content of your beliefs.
- If your hurt is non-ego-based, either take your awfulizing belief and your non-awfulizing belief or your discomfort intolerance belief and discomfort tolerance belief and question the relevant pairing by again asking the same three questions as above, providing reasons for your answers as before. See Appendices 4 and 5 for suggestions concerning arguments on this issue, which have to be tailored to the content of your beliefs.
- In addition, if you held a self-pity belief you can take this (e.g. 'My friends neglected me. Poor me!') and the healthy, non-self-pity belief alternative (e.g. 'My friends neglected me. I am a non-poor person who has been treated poorly') and question these two beliefs.

Having completed this process you should understand why your IBs are irrational and why the rational alternatives to these beliefs are rational, and will be in a position to commit yourself to act and think in ways consistent with your RBs to enable you to deal effectively with the undeserved bad treatment and/or relationship devaluation about which you made yourself feel hurt.

Face your hurt-related theme in imagery

Assuming you've committed to act on your RBs (i.e. flexible belief and non-extreme belief), you must face up to others treating you badly (where you think you don't deserve such treatment) and relationship devaluation (where someone indicates that his or her relationship with you is less important to him or her than the relationship is to you) and learn to think rationally about it.

Until now you've worked at a general level with respect to your hurt-related theme, dealing with the IBs that account for your hurt and developing your alternative RBs. However, to apply your general RBs in dealing with others treating you badly (where you think you do not deserve such treatment) and with relationship devaluation (where someone indicates that his or her relationship with you is less important to him or her than the relationship is to you), you must remember that since you make yourself hurt about specific events (actual or imagined), you should deal with these by rehearsing specific variants of your RBs.

The best way to do this is in specific situations where others treat you badly (where you think you don't deserve such treatment) and where your relationship is devalued (where someone indicates that his or her relationship with you is less important to him or her than the relationship is to you), but you may benefit by first using imagery as follows:

- Imagine a specific situation in which you felt hurt or may feel hurt about
  - others treating you badly (where you think you don't deserve such treatment); or
  - where someone indicates that his or her relationship with you is less important to him or her than the relationship is to you, and focus, in your mind's eye, on what you felt most hurt about (i.e. your 'A').
- Focusing on 'A' while rehearsing a specific and relevant RB, try to make yourself feel sorrowful but not hurt.
- Imagine yourself acting in ways consistent with your RB, e.g. expressing your sorrow, asking the other person for his or her perspective and engaging the other person in a productive dialogue.
- Recognize that some of your post-belief thinking may be distorted. Respond without getting bogged down doing so. Accept the presence of any remaining distorted thoughts without engaging with them.
- Repeat these steps until you feel ready to put this sequence into practice in your life.

Face those who have treated you unfairly or who have devalued your relationship with them

Once you've got yourself into a rational frame of mind concerning a situation about which you felt hurt, so that you now feel sorrowful about it, you're in a position to tell people how you healthily feel about what they did or didn't do. As you do so, don't blame them for the feelings of hurt you initially felt when you held IBs about their behaviour or its lack. Once you do this, be ready to listen to their response and try to understand them from their perspective. If you do so, they may well let go of their defensiveness and also may – I stress the word *may* – apologize for their behaviour. However, even if they don't apologize, once you hold RBs about their unfair behaviour (for example) rather than IBs, you have more of a chance of having a constructive dialogue over the episode and of coming to a constructive resolution.

Capitalize on what you have learned and generalize your learning

When you've faced your hurt and dealt with it as best you can, reflect on what you did and what you learned. In particular, if you were able to face the person you previously thought had hurt you, and could rehearse your specific RBs and take constructive action, then ask yourself how you could capitalize on what you achieved and generalize your learning to similar or different hurt-related situations.

Deal with any problems facing hurt-related situations

If you experienced problems facing the person who treated you badly and undeservedly or who devalued his or her relationship with you using the above steps, answer the following:

- Did I face the hurt-related situation. If not, why not?
- Did I rehearse my RBs before and during facing the hurt-related situation? If not, why not?
- Did I execute my plan to face the hurt-related situation? If not, why not?
- Did I engage with post-belief distorted thinking? If so, why?

Reflect on your experience and put into practice what you have learned next time you face the hurt-related situation.

Become less hurt-prone

So far I've discussed how you can help yourself deal with hurt about specified occasions where the other person treated you badly and undeservedly or devalued his or her relationship with you. However, if you're particularly hurt-prone (i.e. you often think others treat you badly and undeservedly and devalue their relationship with you and you feel hurt about this), do the following.

Accept yourself unconditionally for being hurt-prone

If you're hurt-prone for whatever reason, you have an important choice to make at the outset: you can accept yourself unconditionally as a fallible human being with a proneness to experiencing hurt or you can depreciate yourself for this proneness. Before making your choice, remember that unconditional self-acceptance doesn't mean you need to resign yourself to a lifetime of hurt-proneness. It means you're a fallible human being whether or not you're hurt-prone. It doesn't indicate that you cannot work to become less hurt-prone. Indeed, it helps you do this. If you depreciate yourself for being hurt-prone, you not only have emotional disturbance stemming from hurt-proneness, you're disturbing yourself about this disturbance: you have two disturbances for the price of one. So accepting yourself unconditionally for your hurt-proneness not only spares you this secondary disturbance but helps you focus on your proneness with the purpose of helping you become less prone.

My advice is: choose to accept yourself unconditionally for being hurt-prone.

Deal with emotional problems about hurt

In the same way that you may disturb yourself about being hurt-prone, you may also disturb yourself about specific instances of hurt. Thus, you may make yourself:

* anxious about the prospect of experiencing hurt;
* depressed about feeling hurt;
* ashamed about feeling hurt; or
* unhealthily angry with yourself for making yourself feel hurt.

See the chapters on anxiety, depression, shame and unhealthy anger for help if you tend to disturb yourself about feeling hurt.

Why you feel hurt much of the time and how to deal with this

If you're particularly hurt-prone, you hold the following belief, which I call a 'chronic hurt-based general IB': 'Once I invest in people close to me, I must get, and see clearly that I'm getting, a fair return on that investment. If I don't it's terrible and proves I'm unworthy or to be pitied.'

Holding this belief will mean you'll do the following:

* You'll often focus on past relationships where others have treated you unfairly or where their investment in your relationship wasn't as strong as yours.
* You scan your current relationships, certain to find evidence that others are treating you badly or that they don't care for you as much as you care for them. If there's any ambiguity about this, you err on the side of undeserved treatment and relationship devaluation.
* Finally, as we've seen, you'll avoid getting close to people because you're sure that, in your terms, they'll hurt you.

How to deal with chronic hurt

To deal with this chronic sense of hurt, you should develop and apply an alternative general RB which protects you from such hurt: 'Once I invest in people close to me, I really want to get, and see clearly that I'm getting, a fair return on that investment, but I don't have to do so. If I don't, it's bad but not terrible, and does not prove that I'm unworthy or to be pitied. Rather, I'm a non-poor, fallible human being who has been treated poorly.'

Such a belief will lead you to think that the following occurred only when there is clear evidence for making such an inference:

- Someone did take advantage of your good nature and treated you unfairly.
- The other person doesn't value your relationship with you as much as you value your relationship with him or her.

When there is such evidence you'll feel sorrow rather than hurt because you'll be processing this with a specific RB.

In addition, this belief will help you think of times in the past when others did treat you fairly and reciprocated your positive feelings about the relationship, and will help you see the potential for good in future relationships as well as the potential for bad.

How to examine the accuracy of your hurt-related inference if necessary

If you're still unsure that people have treated you badly or do not reciprocate the value you put on your relationship with them, answer one or more of the following questions:

- How valid is my inference that the other person has betrayed me (for example)?
- Would an objective jury agree that the other person has betrayed me? If not, what would their verdict be?
- Is my inference that the other person has betrayed me realistic? If not, what is a more realistic inference?
- If I asked someone I could trust to give me an objective opinion about my inference that the other person has betrayed me, what would he or she say to me and why? What inference would he or she encourage me to make instead?
- If a friend had told me she had made the same inference about being betrayed in the same situation, what would I say to her about the validity of her inference and why? What inference would I encourage her to make instead?

Understand the thinking consequences of your IBs

When you hold a set of IBs about undeserved bad treatment and relationship devaluation then, as discussed, a consequence is that your subsequent thinking is highly distorted and skewed to the negative.

If you don't understand how your mind works in this respect, you'll get caught up in your compelling distorted thoughts and will regard them as representing reality and will thus strive to protect yourself from what you regard as real negative events, rather than seeing them as highly distorted thinking consequences of IBs you've created.

However, if you do understand this phenomenon and act on this understanding, you'll trace such thinking back to the IBs that spawned it and will do one of two things (or both):

* question these IBs;
* acknowledge the existence of such distorted thinking and go about your business while neither engaging with it nor trying to eliminate it; you'll maintain this understanding no matter how compelling your distorted thoughts are.

Adopt a healthy orientation towards reciprocity in close relationships and its absence

Developing a healthy orientation towards reciprocity in relationships and, in particular, its absence is an important part of becoming less hurt-prone. This involves you doing the following:

* Recognize that there's nothing intrinsically wrong with wanting reciprocity in relationships. However, it's also important to acknowledge that what you want from a relationship with a person may not be the same as what that person wants from a relationship with you.
* Recognize that most of the time when you act fairly towards others, they'll act fairly towards you, i.e. fair treatment tends to yield fair treatment. However, this is certainly not a universal rule and sometimes people close to you will take advantage of your good nature and betray your trust and otherwise treat you unfairly. It's important that you don't add disturbance to this adversity by demanding that the reciprocity effect must exist in such situations. It doesn't, and no amount of demanding that it must will make it so. Rather, look at the situation from your rational flexible and non-extreme mind. When you do so you'll still feel very badly about it (i.e. sorrow), but you won't be disturbed (i.e. hurt).

Summary

You can make yourself less hurt-prone by:

- accepting yourself unconditionally for being hurt-prone;
- dealing effectively with your emotional problems about hurt;
- developing a flexible attitude towards reciprocity in relationships and a realistic view when this reciprocity is absent;
- understanding that when you hold IBs about undeserved bad treatment and relationship devaluation, you exaggerate the nature of these inferences and its consequences. However, you will not engage with such thinking but will trace it back to the IBs that spawned it, which you will challenge; you will then let any remnants of such thinking be, again without engaging with it or trying to eliminate it.

In the next chapter, I deal with the deadly emotion known as unhealthy anger.

7

Dealing with unhealthy anger

This chapter outlines the RECBT view of unhealthy anger and its healthy alternative, healthy anger, showing how to deal effectively with this deadly emotion.

Understanding unhealthy anger

This section discusses the RECBT view of what happens when you make yourself unhealthily angry and how to deal effectively with this deadly emotion, using RECBT's 'ABC' model where 'A' stands for 'adversity', 'B' for beliefs and 'C' for the consequences of these beliefs. However, I will use the order 'CAB' since it's best to start with features of unhealthy anger at 'C'.

'C'

Chapter 1 explained that there are three main features of any emotional problem: feeling, behavioural and thinking. You're likely to feel unhealthily angry in several ways. Common experiences include marked increase in heart rate, feeling hot and bothered, feeling very agitated and as if you want to explode. Your mind tends to race and you can't think straight. These feelings tend to interfere with your thinking clearly about what you feel unhealthily angry about and impede constructive action.

Behaviour associated with unhealthy anger

When feeling unhealthily angry, you tend to act as outlined in Table 7.1.

Thinking associated with unhealthy anger

When you feel unhealthily angry, you tend to think as outlined in Table 7.1, exaggerating what you originally felt unhealthily jealous about and see as its likely consequences.

'A'

Chapter 1 explained that 'A' stands for adversity: what you're most disturbed about with respect to your personal domain. When feeling

Table 7.1 Unhealthy anger vs healthy anger

Adversity	• You think that you have been frustrated in some way.	
	• Your movement towards an important goal has been obstructed in some way.	
	• Someone has transgressed one of your personal rules.	
	• You have transgressed one of your own personal rules.	
	• Someone has disrespected you.	
	• Someone or something has threatened your self-esteem.	

Belief	**IRRATIONAL**	**RATIONAL**
Emotion	**Unhealthy anger**	**Healthy anger**
Behaviour	• You attack the other(s) physically. • You attack the other(s) verbally. • You attack the other(s) passive-aggressively. • You displace the attack on to another person, animal or object. • You withdraw aggressively. • You recruit allies against the other(s).	• You assert yourself with the other(s). • You request, but do not demand, behavioural change from the other(s). • You express your feelings about the loss, failure or undeserved plight and talk in a non-complaining way about your feelings about these to significant others. • You leave an unsatisfactory situation non-aggressively after taking steps to deal with it.
Subsequent thinking	• You overestimate the extent to which the other(s) acted deliberately. • You see malicious intent in the motives of the other(s). • You see yourself as definitely right and the other(s) as definitely wrong. • You are unable to see the point of view of the other(s). • You plot to exact revenge. • You ruminate about the other's behaviour and imagine coming out on top.	• You think that the other(s) may have acted deliberately, but you also recognize that this may not have been the case. • You are able to see the point of view of the other(s). • You have fleeting rather than sustained thoughts to exact revenge. • You think that the other(s) may have had malicious intent in their motives, but you also recognize that this may not have been the case. • You think that you are probably rather than definitely right, and the other(s) are probably rather than definitely wrong.

unhealthily jealous, you make one or more of the following inferences. You think that:

• you have been frustrated in some way;
• your movement towards an important goal has been obstructed in some way;
• someone has transgressed one of your personal rules;
• you've transgressed one of your own personal rules;
• someone has disrespected you;
• someone or something has threatened your self-esteem.

As with other deadly emotions discussed in this book, perhaps with the exception of shame and guilt, these inferences related to unhealthy anger may occur in either the ego realm or the non-ego realm of your personal domain.

'B'

As Chapter 1 explained, beliefs are at the heart of the RECBT model of the emotions. Anger-related inferences, on their own, don't explain your unhealthy anger, since, as I show, it's possible and desirable to feel healthily angry about these inferences. As Chapter 1 indicated, you can hold a set of IBs or RBs about adversity.

IBs about frustration/goal obstruction/rule transgression/disrespect or self-esteem threat

The RECBT model of unhealthy anger is that you feel unhealthily angry about being frustrated; having your goals obstructed; someone (including yourself) transgressing your personal rules; and someone disrespecting you or threatening your self-esteem when you hold IBs about these inferences. These beliefs are rigid and extreme. Please note:

• rigid beliefs are common to both ego unhealthy anger and non-ego unhealthy anger;
• self-depreciation beliefs are the main extreme beliefs in ego unhealthy anger;
• other-depreciation beliefs can occur in both ego unhealthy anger and non-ego unhealthy anger;
• awfulizing beliefs and discomfort intolerance beliefs also occur in non-ego unhealthy anger.

Understanding healthy anger

As Chapter 1 explained, when you face a negative event it's healthy to experience a negative emotion that helps you deal effectively with the negative event you face. This section discusses the RECBT view of healthy anger as the healthy alternative to unhealthy anger, again using the 'CABDE' order of the 'ABCDE' framework.

'C'

As explained above, there are three main features of unhealthy anger: feeling, behavioural and thinking. The same is true when you're healthily angry rather than unhealthily angry. Common experiences include an increase in heart rate (though perhaps not as marked as in unhealthy anger), feeling warm rather than hot and bothered, and not feeling as if you want to explode. Perhaps the main difference in this respect is that while your mind tends to race and you can't think straight in unhealthy anger, your mind tends to be more focused in healthy anger and you can think more clearly. Such feelings in healthy anger tend to motivate you to take constructive action.

Behaviour associated with healthy anger

When healthily rather than unhealthily angry, you're motivated to face the frustration or obstacle to goal progress and deal with this in a thoughtful, problem-solving manner. If another person has transgressed your rule, disrespected you or otherwise threatened your self-esteem, you're motivated to assert yourself with that person in a clear but respectful manner. Table 7.1 outlines the major ways you act or feel like acting when healthily angry.

Thinking associated with healthy anger

When healthily rather than unhealthily angry, you tend to think in ways designed to help you face and deal effectively with the situations detailed above (see Table 7.1).

'A'

When healthily angry, what you feel healthily angry about is the same as you feel unhealthily angry about (see Table 7.1). You think that:

- you've been frustrated in some way;
- your movement towards an important goal has been obstructed in some way;
- someone has transgressed one of your personal rules;
- you've transgressed one of your own personal rules;
- someone has disrespected you;
- someone or something has threatened your self-esteem.

'B'

When you feel healthily rather than unhealthily angry about one or more of the above anger-related inferences, you do so because the beliefs you hold about these inferences are rational.

RBs about frustration/goal obstruction/rule transgression/disrespect or self-esteem threat

The RECBT model of healthy anger is that you feel healthily angry about the above anger-related inferences when you hold RBs about these inferences. These beliefs are flexible and non-extreme. Please note:

- flexible beliefs are common to both ego healthy anger and non-ego healthy anger;
- unconditional self-acceptance beliefs are the main non-extreme beliefs in ego healthy anger;
- unconditional other-acceptance beliefs can occur in both ego healthy anger and non-ego healthy anger;
- non-awfulizing beliefs and discomfort tolerance beliefs also occur in non-ego healthy anger.

How to deal with unhealthy anger

Since you make yourself unhealthily angry about frustration/goal obstruction/rule transgression/ disrespect or threats to self-esteem, your goal is to make yourself healthily angry rather than unhealthily angry about these same inferences. That's why I'll be encouraging you to assume temporarily that your inferences of frustration/goal obstruction/rule transgression/ disrespect or threats to self-esteem at 'A' are correct. Once you're healthily rather than unhealthily angry, you'll be in a sufficiently rational frame of mind to examine your anger-related inferences. If you're unhealthily angry about these inferences, you won't be objective enough while examining them. Later, I'll explain why you're prone to inferring the existence of such inferences in ambiguous situations and will help you become less prone.

Ensure that you're feeling unhealthily angry and it's a problem for you

Before doing anything to try to change your feelings of unhealthy anger, ensure that you're unhealthily angry and that you see unhealthy anger is a problem for you. Otherwise, you'll resist your own efforts to help yourself.

Do you feel unhealthily angry?

People use the term 'anger' loosely; if you say you feel angry, you may or may not be experiencing the deadly version of this emotion. Determine whether you're experiencing the deadly version by consulting the behavioural and thinking consequences of both IBs and RBs about anger-related inferences. The more your behaviour and thinking match those listed in Table 7.1 as consequences of IBs, the more likely you feel/felt unhealthily angry rather than healthily angry. Conversely, the more your behaviour and thinking match those listed as consequences of RBs, the more likely you feel/felt healthily angry rather than unhealthily angry.

Is unhealthy anger a problem for you?

Assuming you've determined that you experienced unhealthy anger rather than healthy anger, now determine whether you consider your unhealthy anger is a problem you want to change. Just because your experience matches those listed in Table 7.1 as unhealthy anger doesn't mean you'll inevitably see it's a problem for you.

If you're uncertain whether unhealthy anger is a problem for you, answer the following:

- Does my unhealthy anger help me deal effectively with frustration, goal obstruction, rule transgression and/or others showing me disrespect or threatening my self-esteem?
- Does my unhealthy anger motivate me to engage relevant others in a productive dialogue?

If you've answered 'yes' to either or both questions, you may be reluctant to target your unhealthy anger for change. I suggest you read the following section with an open mind, then answer two different questions.

Commit to healthy anger as a productive alternative to unhealthy anger

In any self-change venture, you need clear alternatives to problems you wish to change. Otherwise you'll be in a 'change vacuum', where you know what you don't want to feel but don't know what it would be healthy for you to feel instead. RECBT argues that when you face (or think you're facing) frustration, goal obstruction, rule transgression, disrespect or a threat to your self-esteem, the healthy alternative to feeling unhealthily angry about these inferences is to feel healthily angry about them. Table 7.1 lists the behavioural and thinking consequences of RBs about these anger-related inferences associated with healthy anger. If you see that these consequences help you deal effectively with these inferences, you're ready to commit yourself to feeling healthily angry rather than unhealthily angry about such inferences.

For those ambivalent about targeting unhealthy anger as a problem to change in the previous section, answer the following questions while consulting the relevant sections of Table 7.1:

- Will unhealthy anger or healthy anger help me deal more effectively with frustration, goal obstruction, rule transgression, disrespect or a threat to my self-esteem?
- Which will help me more to engage relevant others in a productive dialogue: unhealthy anger or healthy anger?

Hopefully, if you were ambivalent about targeting your unhealthy anger for change, you're now ready to do so and to work towards feeling healthily rather than unhealthily angry about frustration, goal obstruction, rule transgression, disrespect or a threat to your self-esteem.

Identify what you're most unhealthily angry about at 'A'

If you have a problem with unhealthy anger, you're likely to experience this deadly emotion in situations where you infer the existence of frustration, goal obstruction, rule transgression, disrespect or a threat to your self-esteem. For our purposes in this chapter, there are two realms of your personal domain:

- the ego realm, where you infer the presence of these situations as impacting on your self-esteem;
- the non-ego realm, where you infer the presence of these situations as impacting on your sense of comfort, broadly defined.

Such inferences can exist in both realms. To identify what you're unhealthily angry about, ask yourself:

- What was I most unhealthily angry about in the situation I was in?
- Did I think I was being frustrated? If so, in what way?
- Did I consider my progress towards an important goal was being obstructed? If so, what was my goal and the nature of the obstruction?
- Did I think that I or someone else transgressed one of my rules? If so, who transgressed the rule, what rule did I/they transgress and how did I/they transgress it?
- Did someone disrespect me? If so, how did they show disrespect for me?
- Did someone or something threaten my self-esteem? If so, what was the nature and source of the threat?

Use the 'magic question' technique

If you still cannot identify your unhealthy anger-related inference, use the 'magic question' technique:

- Focus on the situation in which you felt unhealthily angry.
- Without changing the situation, ask yourself: 'What one thing would have eliminated or significantly reduced my unhealthy anger?'
- The opposite is what you were most unhealthily angry about.

Here's how Serge used this technique:

- I felt unhealthily angry when my daughter went out without saying goodbye to me.
- If I'd known she hadn't disrespected me, I wouldn't have felt unhealthily angry.
- I was most unhealthily angry about my daughter disrespecting me by leaving without saying goodbye.

Identify the IBs underpinning your unhealthy anger and the rational alternatives underpinning healthy anger

The RECBT model argues that frustration, goal obstruction, rule transgression, disrespect and threats to your self-esteem don't make you feel unhealthily angry. Rather, you make yourself unhealthily angry by holding IBs (at 'B') about these inferences, and if you hold RBs (also at 'B') about them instead you'll feel healthy rather than unhealthy anger.

Consequently, you should identify your IBs about your anger-related inferences at 'A' and the rational alternatives to these IBs. I recommend the latter so you can derive hope that you can see there's an alternative to the main determining factor of your unhealthy anger.

In identifying your IBs and alternative RBs, determine whether your unhealthy anger is ego-related, impacting on your self-esteem, or non-ego-related, impacting on your sense of comfort, broadly defined, and not impacting on your self-esteem. Then do the following.

Ego unhealthy anger

If your unhealthy anger is ego-related, identify your rigid belief and either your self-depreciation belief or other-depreciation belief about what you were most unhealthily angry about at 'A'. Then identify their rational alternatives, i.e. your flexible belief and unconditional self-acceptance or unconditional other-acceptance belief.

Non-ego unhealthy anger

If your unhealthy anger is non-ego-related, identify your rigid belief and either your awfulizing belief, your discomfort intolerance belief or your other-depreciation belief about what you were most unhealthily angry about at 'A'. Then identify their rational alternatives, i.e. your flexible belief and either your non-awfulizing belief, your discomfort tolerance belief or your unconditional other-acceptance belief.

Acknowledge the 'B–C' connection

Before proceeding to question these beliefs, acknowledge the connection between your IBs (at 'B') and your unhealthy anger (at 'C') and between your RBs (at 'B') and healthy anger (at 'E') that you're aiming to experience in response to your anger-related inference (at 'A').

Question your beliefs

You're now ready to question your beliefs to see clearly that your IBs are irrational (i.e. false, illogical and largely unhelpful) and that your alternative RBs are rational (i.e. true, logical and largely helpful). To enable you to get the most out of this process:

- Begin by questioning your rigid belief and flexible belief together. Ask yourself:
  - Which of these beliefs is true? Which is false?
  - Which of these beliefs is logical? Which is illogical?
  - Which of these beliefs is largely helpful? Which is largely unhelpful?
  Provide reasons for your answers. See Appendix 2 for suggestions concerning arguments on this issue. You'll need to tailor your arguments to the content of your beliefs.
- If your unhealthy anger is ego-based, take your self-depreciation belief or other-depreciation belief and unconditional self-acceptance belief or unconditional other-acceptance belief and question them by asking the same three questions as above. Again provide reasons for your answers. See Appendix 3 for suggestions concerning arguments on this issue, which have to be tailored to the content of your beliefs.
- If your unhealthy anger is non-ego-based, take either your awfulizing belief and non-awfulizing belief, discomfort intolerance belief and discomfort tolerance belief or other-depreciation belief and unconditional other-acceptance belief and question the relevant pairing by asking the same three questions as above, providing reasons for your answers as before. See Appendices 3, 4 and 5 for suggestions concerning arguments on this issue, which again have to be tailored to the content of your beliefs.

Having completed this questioning process you should understand why your IBs are irrational and why the rational alternatives to these beliefs are rational, and you should be in a position to commit yourself to act and think in ways consistent with your RBs to enable you to deal effectively with whatever it was you were unhealthily angry about in the first instance.

Face your unhealthy anger-related theme in imagery

Assuming you've committed to act on your RBs (flexible belief and non-extreme belief), you must face up to what you were most unhealthily angry about and learn to think rationally about it.

Until now you've worked generally in regard to your unhealthy anger-related inference, the IBs that account for your unhealthy anger and developing your alternative RBs. However, to apply your RBs in dealing with this inference, remember that since you make yourself unhealthily angry about specific events (actual or imagined), you should deal with these by rehearsing specific variants of your RBs.

The best way to do this is in specific situations in which you made yourself unhealthily angry, but you may benefit by first using imagery as follows:

- Imagine a specific situation in which you felt unhealthily angry or may feel unhealthily angry about frustration, goal obstruction, rule transgression, disrespect or a threat to your self-esteem; focus mentally on what you felt most unhealthily angry about (i.e. your 'A').
- Focusing on 'A' while rehearsing a specific RB, try to make yourself feel healthily angry, but not unhealthily angry.
- Imagine yourself acting in ways consistent with your RB, e.g. asserting yourself with the other person and engaging him or her in productive dialogue.
- Recognize that some of your post-belief thinking may be distorted. Respond without getting bogged down doing so. Accept the presence of any remaining distorted thoughts without engaging with them.
- Repeat the above steps until you feel ready to put this sequence into practice in your life.

Act assertively in relevant anger-related situations

Whether or not you've used imagery as a preparatory step, you need to take the following steps when you assert yourself in anger-related situations.

- Choose a specific situation containing the theme about which you're likely to make yourself unhealthily angry.
- Make a plan of how you're going to assert yourself in the situation.
- Rehearse a specific version of your general RBs before entering the situation so you can face what you're angry about in a rational frame of mind. It would also be useful to develop a shorthand version of your specific RB to use in the situation.
- Enter the situation, accepting the fact that you're likely to be uncomfortable doing so. Assert yourself as previously planned. React to any consequences from a rational frame of mind if you can.

- Recognize that even though you've got yourself into a rational frame of mind, some of your thinking may be distorted and unrealistic; some may be realistic and balanced. Accept the presence of the former and don't engage with it. Engage with the latter as much as you can.

Capitalize on what you learned and generalize your learning

When you've faced the person, for example, and asserted yourself with him or her as best you could, reflect on what you did and what you learned. In particular, if you were able to (1) face the person, (2) rehearse your specific RBs and (3) assert yourself, ask yourself how you can capitalize on what you achieved and generalize your learning to similar or different unhealthy anger-related situations.

Deal with any problems facing unhealthy anger-related situations

If you experienced any problems facing the person with whom you were unhealthily angry using the above steps, answer the following:

- Did I face the person? If not, why not?
- Did I rehearse my RBs before and during facing the person? If not, why not?
- Did I engage with post-belief distorted thinking? If so, why?

Reflect on your experience and put into practice what you have learned for the next time you face the unhealthy anger-related situation.

Become less prone to unhealthy anger

So far I've discussed how you can help yourself deal with unhealthy anger about specified occasions where you've been frustrated, experienced an obstruction towards pursuing a valued goal, where someone (including yourself) has transgressed one of your rules or someone has disrespected you or threatened your self-esteem. However, what if you're particularly prone to unhealthy anger (i.e. you often think you've been frustrated, that your goals are being obstructed, your rules are being transgressed, others have disrespected you or threatened your self-esteem and you feel unhealthily angry about this)? I suggest you do the following.

Accept yourself unconditionally for being prone to unhealthy anger

If you're prone to unhealthy anger, for whatever reason, you have an important choice to make at the outset: you can accept yourself unconditionally as a fallible human being, prone to experiencing unhealthy anger, or you can depreciate yourself for this proneness. Before making your choice, remember that unconditional self-acceptance doesn't mean you need to resign yourself to a lifetime of proneness to unhealthy anger. It means you're a fallible human being, whether or not prone to unhealthy anger. It doesn't indicate that you cannot work to become less prone to this deadly emotion. Indeed, it helps you do this. If you depreciate yourself for being prone to unhealthy anger, you not only have emotional disturbance stemming from unhealthy anger-proneness, you're also disturbing yourself about this disturbance: two disturbances for the price of one. So accepting yourself unconditionally for your proneness to unhealthy anger not only spares you this secondary disturbance but helps you focus on your proneness with the purpose of helping yourself become less prone.

My advice then is: choose to accept yourself unconditionally for being prone to unhealthy anger.

Deal with emotional problems about unhealthy anger

Just as you may disturb yourself about being prone to unhealthy anger, you may also disturb yourself about specific instances of unhealthy anger by making yourself:

- anxious about the prospect of experiencing unhealthy anger;
- depressed about feeling unhealthily angry;
- guilty about feeling unhealthily angry;
- ashamed about feeling unhealthily angry; or
- unhealthily angry with yourself for making yourself unhealthily angry.

See the chapters on anxiety, depression, guilt and shame for help if you tend to disturb yourself about feeling unhealthily angry.

Assessing unhealthy self-anger about unhealthy anger

When you're unhealthily angry with yourself about your unhealthy anger, you clearly think you've broken your own rule about experiencing unhealthy anger. This may be about the whole response itself or one or more of its components (i.e. the feeling, behavioural or thinking component). In my experience, you're most likely to be unhealthily angry with yourself for what you did (or felt like doing) when you were originally unhealthily angry.

Dealing with unhealthy self-anger about unhealthy anger

Unless you deal with your unhealthy self-anger about unhealthy anger, you're unlikely to deal with your original unhealthy anger because your focus will be on blaming yourself for your anger problem, which will take you away from dealing with this problem.

The best way of dealing with your unhealthy self-anger about your original unhealthy anger is to accept yourself unconditionally for having a problem with unhealthy anger. Yes, you may be breaking one of your personal rules by being unhealthily angry and expressing it in unconstructive ways, but sadly there's no reason why you mustn't break your rule about being or expressing your unhealthy anger. You're human, and humans do break their rules. That doesn't mean you shouldn't take responsibility for making yourself unhealthily angry in the first place and expressing it unconstructively in the second place. Unless you take responsibility for your unhealthy anger, you won't deal with it. But you can take responsibility without the self-blame that's a central feature of your unhealthy self-anger about your original anger problem.

Why you feel unhealthily angry much of the time and how to deal with this

If you're particularly prone to unhealthy anger, you tend to make anger-related inferences in ambiguous situations. I'll explain this by using disrespect inferences as an example. When you're prone to unhealthy anger you hold a general IB such as: 'It must be clear that the other person hasn't shown me disrespect. I can't bear such ambiguity.'

Holding this belief means that you'll assume the other person has shown you disrespect if you're not convinced he or she hasn't; then you'll make yourself unhealthily angry about this inferred disrespect.

How to deal with chronic unhealthy anger

To deal with chronic unhealthy anger, develop and apply an alternative general RB, e.g. 'It would be good if I were clear that the other person hasn't shown me disrespect, but I don't need it. Not having it is difficult to tolerate, but I can do so and it's worth it to me to do so.'

Such a belief will lead you to think that the other person has disrespected you only where there's clear evidence for making such an inference. When there is, you need to hold a specific RB about such disrespect.

How to examine the accuracy of anger-related inference if necessary

If you're still unsure whether your inference of disrespect is accurate or inaccurate, answer one or more of the following questions:

- How likely is it that I was disrespected (or might be disrespected)?
- Would an objective jury agree that I was (or might be) disrespected? If not, what would their verdict be?
- Did I view (am I viewing) the situation in which I inferred disrespect realistically? If not, how could I have viewed (can I view) it more realistically?
- If I asked someone I could trust to give me an objective opinion about

the truth or falsity of my inference about being disrespected, what would that person say to me and why? What inference would he or she encourage me to make instead?
- If a friend told me he faced (or was about to face) the same situation as I faced and had made the same inference of disrespect, what would I say to him about the validity of his inference and why? What inference would I encourage him to make instead?

Understand the thinking consequences of your IBs

When you hold a set of IBs about frustration/goal obstruction/rule transgression/disrespect and a threat to your self-esteem, as discussed, a consequence is that your subsequent thinking is highly distorted and skewed to the negative.

If you don't understand how your mind works in this respect, you'll get caught up in your compelling distorted thoughts, regard them as representing reality and strive to protect yourself from what you regard as real negative events rather than seeing them as highly distorted thinking consequences of IBs you've created.

However, if you do understand this phenomenon and act on this understanding, you'll trace such thinking back to the IBs that spawned it and will do one of two things (or both):

- question these IBs;
- acknowledge the existence of such distorted thinking and go about your business, neither engaging with it nor trying to eliminate it; you'll maintain this understanding no matter how compelling your distorted thoughts are.

Summary

You can make yourself less prone to unhealthy anger by:

- accepting yourself unconditionally for being prone to unhealthy anger;
- dealing effectively with your emotional problems about unhealthy anger;
- developing RBs enabling you to make realistic inferences at 'A';
- understanding that when you hold IBs about frustration/goal obstruction/rule transgression/disrespect or threats to your self-esteem, you'll exaggerate the nature of these inferences and its consequences. However, you will not engage with such thinking but trace it back to the IBs that spawned it, which you'll challenge; you'll then let any remnants of such thinking be, again without engaging with it or trying to eliminate it.

In the next chapter, I deal with the deadly emotion known as unhealthy jealousy.

8

Dealing with unhealthy jealousy

This chapter outlines the RECBT view of unhealthy jealousy and its healthy alternative, healthy jealousy, showing how to deal effectively with this deadly emotion.

Understanding unhealthy jealousy

This section discusses the RECBT view of what happens when you make yourself unhealthily jealous[6] and how to deal effectively with this deadly emotion, using RECBT's 'ABC' model where 'A' stands for 'adversity', 'B' for beliefs and 'C' for the consequences of these beliefs. However, I will use the order 'CAB' since it's best to start with features of unhealthy jealousy at 'C'.

'C'

Chapter 1 explained that there are three main features of any emotional problem: feeling, behavioural and thinking. You're likely to feel unhealthily jealous in several ways. Common experiences include anxiety, hurt, unhealthy anger and a heightened sense of suspiciousness. These feelings tend to interfere with your thinking clearly about what you feel unhealthily jealous about and impede constructive action.

Behaviour associated with unhealthy jealousy

When feeling unhealthily jealous, you tend to act as outlined in Table 8.1.

Thinking associated with unhealthy jealousy

When you feel unhealthily jealous, you tend to think as outlined in Table 8.1, exaggerating what you originally felt unhealthily jealous about and what you see as its likely consequences.

---

6 Jealousy can be present in a variety of relationships but is most common in romantic relationships. In this chapter, I focus on romantic jealousy.

Table 8.1 Unhealthy jealousy vs healthy jealousy

Adversity	• A threat is posed to your relationship with your partner from a third person. • A threat is posed by uncertainty you face concerning your partner's whereabouts, behaviour or thinking in the context of the first threat.	
Belief	IRRATIONAL	RATIONAL
Emotion	Unhealthy jealousy	Healthy jealousy
Behaviour	• You seek constant reassurance that you are loved. • You monitor the actions and feelings of your partner. • You search for evidence that your partner is involved with someone else. • You attempt to restrict the movements or activities of your partner. • You set tests which your partner has to pass. • You retaliate for your partner's presumed infidelity. • You sulk.	• You allow your partner to initiate expressing love for you without prompting him or her or seeking reassurance once he or she has done so. • You allow your partner freedom without monitoring his or her feelings, actions and whereabouts. • You allow your partner to show natural interest in members of the opposite sex without setting tests.
Subsequent thinking	• You exaggerate any threat to your relationship that does exist. • You think the loss of your relationship is imminent. • You misconstrue your partner's ordinary conversations with relevant others as having romantic or sexual connotations. • You construct visual images of your partner's infidelity. • If your partner admits to finding another person attractive, you think that he or she finds that person more attractive than you and will leave you for this other person.	• You tend not to exaggerate any threat to your relationship that does exist. • You do not misconstrue ordinary conversations between your partner and other men or women. • You do not construct visual images of your partner's infidelity. • You accept that your partner will find others attractive but you do not see this as a threat.

'A'

Chapter 1 explained that 'A' stands for adversity: what you're most disturbed about with respect to your personal domain. When you feel unhealthily jealous, you make one or more of the following inferences. You think that:

- a threat is posed from a third person to your relationship with your partner;
- a threat is posed by the uncertainty you face concerning your partner's whereabouts, behaviour, thoughts and feelings in the context of the first threat.[7]

As with other deadly emotions discussed in this book, perhaps with the exception of shame and guilt, these unhealthy jealousy-related inferences may occur in either the ego realm or the non-ego realm of your personal domain.

'B'

As Chapter 1 explained, beliefs are at the heart of the RECBT model of the emotions. Jealousy-related inferences, on their own, don't explain your unhealthy jealousy, since, as I show, it's possible and desirable to feel healthily jealous about these inferences. Chapter 1 indicated that you can hold a set of IBs or RBs about adversity.

IBs about relationship and uncertainty threats

The RECBT model of unhealthy jealousy is that you feel unhealthily jealous about the existence of a threat to your relationship and/or uncertainty about your partner's whereabouts when you hold IBs about these inferences. These beliefs are rigid and extreme. Please note:

- rigid beliefs are common to both ego unhealthy jealousy and non-ego unhealthy jealousy;
- self-depreciation beliefs are the main extreme beliefs in ego unhealthy jealousy;
- other-depreciation beliefs can occur in both ego unhealthy jealousy and non-ego unhealthy jealousy;
- awfulizing beliefs and discomfort intolerance beliefs also occur in non-ego unhealthy jealousy.

---

7 In this chapter the term 'whereabouts' includes your partner's behaviour, thoughts and feelings.

Understanding healthy jealousy

As Chapter 1 explained, when you face a negative event it's healthy to experience a negative emotion that helps you deal effectively with the negative event you face. This section discusses the RECBT view of healthy jealousy as the healthy alternative to unhealthy jealousy, again using the 'CABDE' order of the 'ABCDE' framework.

'C'

As explained above, there are three main features of unhealthy jealousy: feeling, behavioural and thinking. The same is true when you're healthily jealous rather than unhealthily jealous. Common experiences include concern, sorrow and healthy anger, but you're not overly suspicious. Such feelings in healthy jealousy help you think more clearly about relationship threats and related uncertainty threats and tend to motivate you to take constructive action.

Behaviour associated with healthy jealousy

When healthily rather than unhealthily jealous, you're motivated to tolerate uncertainty and discuss your concerns with your partner in an open-minded manner. Table 8.1 outlines the major ways you act or feel like acting when healthily jealous.

Thinking associated with healthy jealousy

When healthily rather than unhealthily jealous, you tend to think in ways designed to help you deal effectively with the threats you think you face (see Table 8.1).

'A'

When healthily jealous, what you feel healthily jealous about is the same as what you feel unhealthily jealous about (see Table 8.1). You think that:

- a threat is posed from a third person to your relationship with your partner;
- a threat is posed by the uncertainty you face concerning your partner's whereabouts, behaviour, thoughts and feelings in the context of the first threat.

'B'

When you feel healthily rather than unhealthily jealous about one or both of the above threats, you do so because the beliefs you hold about these inferences are rational.

RBs about relationship threats and related uncertainty threats

The RECBT model of healthy jealousy is that you feel healthily jealous about relationship threats and/or related uncertainty threats when you hold RBs about these inferences. These beliefs are flexible and non-extreme. Please note:

- flexible beliefs are common to both ego healthy jealousy and non-ego healthy jealousy;
- unconditional self-acceptance beliefs are the main non-extreme beliefs in ego healthy jealousy;
- unconditional other-acceptance beliefs can occur in both ego healthy jealousy and non-ego healthy jealousy;
- non-awfulizing beliefs and discomfort tolerance beliefs also occur in non-ego healthy jealousy.

How to deal with unhealthy jealousy

Since you make yourself unhealthily jealous about relationship threats and/or related uncertainty threats, your goal is to make yourself healthily jealous rather than unhealthily jealous about these same inferences. That's why I'll be encouraging you to assume temporarily that your inferences that you're facing a threat to your relationship and/or a related uncertainty threat about your partner's whereabouts at 'A' are correct. Once you're healthily rather than unhealthily jealous, you'll be in a sufficiently rational frame of mind to examine your jealousy-related inferences. If you're unhealthily jealous about these inferences, you won't be objective enough while examining them. Later, I'll explain why you're prone to inferring the existence of such inferences in ambiguous situations and will help you become less prone.

Ensure that you're feeling unhealthily jealous and it's a problem for you

Before doing anything to try to change your feelings of unhealthy jealousy, ensure that you are unhealthily jealous and that you see unhealthy jealousy is a problem for you. Otherwise, you'll resist your own efforts to help yourself.

Do you feel unhealthily jealous?

People use the term 'jealousy' loosely; if you say you feel jealous, you may or may not be experiencing the deadly version of this emotion. Indeed, you may be experiencing envy (discussed in Chapter 9) since people often refer to envy as jealousy. Determine whether you're experiencing the deadly version of jealousy by consulting the behavioural and thinking consequences of both IBs and RBs about jealousy-related inferences. The more your behaviour and thinking match those listed in Table 8.1 as consequences of IBs, the more likely you feel/felt unhealthily jealous, rather than healthily jealous. Conversely, the more your behaviour and thinking match those listed as consequences of RBs, the more likely you feel/felt healthily jealous rather than unhealthily jealous.

Is unhealthy jealousy a problem for you?

Assuming you've determined that you experienced unhealthy jealousy rather than healthy jealousy, now determine whether you consider your unhealthy jealousy is a problem you want to change. Just because your experience matches those listed in Table 8.1 as unhealthy jealousy doesn't mean you'll inevitably see that it's a problem for you.

If you're uncertain whether unhealthy jealousy is a problem for you, answer the following:

• Does my unhealthy jealousy help me deal effectively with relationship threats and/or related uncertainty threats?
• Does my unhealthy jealousy improve or impair my relationship with my partner?
• Does my unhealthy jealousy motivate me to engage my partner in a productive dialogue?

If you've answered 'yes' to one or more of these questions, you may be reluctant to target your unhealthy jealousy for change. I suggest you read the following section with an open mind, then answer three different questions.

Commit to healthy jealousy as a productive alternative to unhealthy jealousy

In any self-change venture, you need clear alternatives to problems you wish to change. Otherwise you'll be in a 'change vacuum', where you know what you don't want to feel but don't know what it would be healthy for you to feel instead. RECBT argues that when you face (or think you're facing) relationship threats and/or related uncertainty threats, the healthy alternative to feeling unhealthily jealous about these inferences is to feel healthily jealous about them. Table 8.1 lists the behavioural and thinking consequences of RBs about these jealousy-related inferences associated with healthy jealousy. If you see that these consequences help you deal effectively with these inferences, you're ready to commit yourself to feeling healthily jealous rather than unhealthily jealous about such inferences.

For those ambivalent about targeting unhealthy jealousy as a problem to change in the previous section, answer the following questions while consulting the relevant sections of Table 8.1:

- Will unhealthy jealousy or healthy jealousy help me deal more effectively with relationship threats and/or related uncertainty threats?
- Which form of jealousy will enhance my relationship with my partner? Which form will impair it?
- Which will help me more to engage my partner in a productive dialogue: unhealthy jealousy or healthy jealousy?

Hopefully, if you were ambivalent about targeting your unhealthy jealousy for change, you're now ready to do so and to work towards feeling healthily rather than unhealthily jealous about relationship threats and/or related uncertainty threats.

Identify what you're most unhealthily jealous about at 'A'

If you have a problem with unhealthy jealousy, you're likely to experience this deadly emotion in situations where you infer the existence of relationship threats and/or related uncertainty threats. For our purposes in this chapter, there are two realms of your personal domain:

- the ego realm, where you infer the presence of these situations as impacting on your self-esteem;
- the non-ego realm, where you infer the presence of these situations as impacting on your sense of comfort, broadly defined.

My experience in counselling people with problems of unhealthy jealousy leads me to conclude that while relationship threats exist in both the ego and non-ego realms of the personal domain, related uncertainty threats tend to exist in the non-ego realm.

To identify what you're unhealthily jealous about, ask yourself:

- What was I most unhealthily jealous about in the situation I was in?
- What threat did I think was being posed to my relationship with my partner?
- Was I facing uncertainty about the whereabouts of my partner?

Use the 'magic question' technique

If you still cannot identify your unhealthy jealousy-related inference, use the 'magic question' technique:

- Focus on the situation in which you felt unhealthily jealous.
- Without changing the situation, ask yourself: 'What one thing would have eliminated or significantly reduced my unhealthy jealousy?'
- The opposite is what you were most unhealthily jealous about.

Here's how Daphne used this technique:

- I felt unhealthily jealous when I saw my partner talking to my boss's wife at the party.
- If I'd known my partner didn't find the boss's wife attractive, I wouldn't have felt unhealthily jealous.
- I was most unhealthily jealous about my partner finding my boss's wife attractive.

Identify the IBs underpinning your unhealthy jealousy and the rational alternatives underpinning healthy jealousy

The RECBT model argues that relationship threats and/or related uncertainty threats don't make you feel unhealthily jealous. Rather, you make yourself unhealthily jealous by holding IBs (at 'B') about these inferences, and if you hold RBs (also at 'B') about them instead you'll feel healthy rather than unhealthy jealousy.

Consequently, you should identify your IBs about your jealousy-related inferences at 'A' and the rational alternatives to these IBs. I recommend the latter so you can derive hope that you can see there's an alternative to the main determining factor of your unhealthy jealousy.

In identifying your IBs and alternative RBs, determine whether your unhealthy jealousy is ego-related, impacting on your self-esteem, or non-ego-related, impacting on your sense of comfort, broadly defined, and not impacting on your self-esteem. Then do the following.

Ego unhealthy jealousy

If your unhealthy jealousy is ego-related, identify your rigid belief and either your self-depreciation belief or other-depreciation belief about what you were most unhealthily jealous about at 'A'. Then identify their rational alternatives, i.e. your flexible belief and unconditional self-acceptance or unconditional other-acceptance belief.

Non-ego unhealthy jealousy

If your unhealthy jealousy is non-ego-related, identify your rigid belief and either your awfulizing belief, your discomfort intolerance belief or your other-depreciation belief about what you were most unhealthily jealous about at 'A'. Then identify their rational alternatives, i.e. your flexible belief and either your non-awfulizing belief, your discomfort tolerance belief or your unconditional other-acceptance belief.

Acknowledge the 'B–C' connection

Before proceeding to question these beliefs, acknowledge the connection between your IBs (at 'B') and unhealthy jealousy (at 'C') and between your RBs (at 'B') and healthy jealousy (at 'E') that you're aiming to experience in response to your jealousy-related inference (at 'A').

Question your beliefs

You're now ready to question your beliefs. The purpose of the questioning process is for you to see clearly that your IBs are irrational (i.e. false, illogical and largely unhelpful) and that your alternative RBs are rational (i.e. true, logical and largely helpful).

To enable you to get the most out of the questioning process:

- Begin by questioning your rigid belief and flexible belief together. Ask yourself:
  - Which of these beliefs is true? Which is false?
  - Which of these beliefs is logical? Which is illogical?
  - Which of these beliefs is largely helpful? Which is largely unhelpful?
  Provide reasons for your answers. See Appendix 2 for suggestions concerning arguments on this issue. You'll need to tailor your arguments to the content of your beliefs.
- If your unhealthy jealousy is ego-based, take your self-depreciation belief or other-depreciation belief and unconditional self-acceptance belief or unconditional other-acceptance belief and question them by asking the same three questions as above. Again provide reasons for your answers. See Appendix 3 for suggestions concerning arguments on this issue, which have to be tailored to the content of your beliefs.
- If your unhealthy jealousy is non-ego-based, take either your awfulizing belief and non-awfulizing belief, discomfort intolerance belief and discomfort tolerance belief or other-depreciation belief and unconditional other-acceptance belief and question the relevant pairing by again asking the same three questions as above, providing reasons for your answers as before. See Appendices 3, 4 and 5 for suggestions concerning arguments on this issue, which again have to be tailored to the content of your beliefs.

Having completed this questioning process you should understand why your IBs are irrational and why the rational alternatives to these beliefs are rational, and you should be in a position to commit yourself to act and think in ways consistent with your RBs to enable you to deal effectively with whatever it was that you were unhealthily jealous about in the first instance.

Face your unhealthy jealousy-related theme in imagery

Assuming you've committed to act on your RBs (flexible belief and non-extreme belief), you must face up to what you were most unhealthily jealous about and learn to think rationally about it.

Until now you've worked generally in regard to your unhealthy jealousy-related inference, the IBs that account for your unhealthy jealousy and developing your alternative RBs. However, to apply your RBs in dealing with this inference, remember that since you make yourself unhealthily jealous about specific events (actual or imagined), you should deal with these by rehearsing specific variants of your RBs.

The best way to do this is in specific situations in which you made yourself unhealthily jealous, but you may benefit by first using imagery as follows:

- Imagine a specific situation in which you felt unhealthily jealous or may feel unhealthily jealous about a relationship threat or a related uncertainty threat; focus mentally on what you felt most unhealthily jealous about (i.e. your 'A').
- Focusing on 'A' while rehearsing a specific RB, try to make yourself feel healthily jealous, but not unhealthily jealous.
- Imagine yourself acting in ways consistent with your RB, e.g. dealing with the uncertainty without questioning your partner or engaging your partner in a productive dialogue if you think it's clear that the threat to your relationship did exist.
- Recognize that some of your post-belief thinking may be distorted. Respond without getting bogged down doing so. Accept the presence of any remaining distorted thoughts without engaging with them.
- Repeat the above steps until you feel ready to put this sequence into practice in your life.

Act and think in ways consistent with your RBs

When you experience the emotional problem of unhealthy jealousy and the thoughts accompanying it, you will also experience a strong urge to act on them. If you do so you'll only serve to strengthen the IBs underpinning such behaviour. So after you've questioned your IBs and RBs as suggested above and committed yourself to strengthening your conviction in your RBs, you should act in ways that will do this and refrain from acting in ways that will do the opposite (see Table 8.1). This is perhaps the most important principle involved in dealing effectively with unhealthy jealousy. I've seen many people in my practice who have had ineffective therapy where the focus was on helping them identify the childhood roots of these feelings. I'm not against this practice, but the reason such therapy often fails is that while the people are engaged in such an exploration they're still acting, in the present, in ways that stem from their IBs and that only serve to reinforce these beliefs.

So it's crucial to act according to behavioural goals you identified earlier and accept that, while you do so, you'll still have the urge to act and think in unhealthy ways. Accept that this is an almost inevitable and natural part of the change process and that these unhealthy urges and thoughts will eventually subside if you don't engage with them. I stress that this is difficult, but if you're clear about what you need to do and act accordingly, you'll stack the odds in favour of, rather than against, dealing effectively with your unhealthy jealousy.

Capitalize on what you have learned and generalize your learning

When you've acted and thought in ways consistent with your RBs, reflect on what you did and what you learned. In particular, if you were able to deal with uncertainty, could rehearse your specific RBs and did nothing to question, check on or monitor your partner, for example, then ask yourself how you can capitalize on what you achieved and generalize your learning to similar or different unhealthy jealousy-related situations.

Deal with any problems facing unhealthy jealousy-related situations

If you experienced any problems facing your unhealthy jealousy situation, answer the following:

- Did I face the situation? If not, why not?
- Did I rehearse my RBs before, during or after facing the situation? If not, why not?
- Did I execute my plan to face the situation? If not, why not?
- Did I engage with post-belief distorted thinking? If so, why?

Reflect on your experience and put into practice what you have learned for next time you face a situation in which someone poses a threat to your relationship, or where a threat is posed by uncertainty concerning your partner's whereabouts, behaviour or thinking in the context of the first threat.

Become less prone to unhealthy jealousy

So far I've discussed how you can help yourself deal with unhealthy jealousy about specified occasions where you faced relationship threats or related uncertainty threats. However, what if you're particularly prone to unhealthy jealousy (i.e. you often think your relationship is under threat and feel unhealthily jealous about this)? I suggest you do the following.

Accept yourself unconditionally for being prone to unhealthy jealousy

If you're prone to unhealthy jealousy for whatever reason, you have an important choice to make at the outset: you can accept yourself uncon-ditionally as a fallible human being, prone to experiencing unhealthy jealousy, or you can depreciate yourself for this proneness. Before making your choice, remember that unconditional self-acceptance doesn't mean you need to resign yourself to a lifetime of proneness to unhealthy jealousy. It means you're a fallible human being, whether or not prone to unhealthy jealousy. It doesn't indicate that you cannot work to become less prone to this deadly emotion. Indeed, it helps you do this. If you depreciate yourself for being prone to unhealthy jealousy, you not only have emotional disturbance stemming from unhealthy jealousy-proneness, you're also disturbing yourself about this disturbance: two disturbances for the price of one. So accepting yourself unconditionally for your proneness to unhealthy jealousy not only spares you this secondary disturbance but helps you focus on your proneness with the purpose of helping yourself become less prone.

My advice then is: choose to accept yourself unconditionally for being prone to unhealthy jealousy.

Deal with emotional problems about unhealthy jealousy

Just as you may disturb yourself about being prone to unhealthy jealousy, you may also disturb yourself about specific instances of unhealthy jealousy by making yourself:

- anxious about the prospect of experiencing unhealthy jealousy;
- depressed about experiencing unhealthy jealousy;
- guilty about experiencing unhealthy jealousy;
- ashamed about or for experiencing unhealthy jealousy;
- unhealthily angry with yourself for making yourself unhealthily jealous.

See the chapters on anxiety, depression, guilt, shame and unhealthy anger for help if you tend to disturb yourself about feeling unhealthily jealous.

Dealing with safety-seeking measures to avoid unhealthy jealousy

I mentioned in Chapter 2 that people use safety-seeking measures to protect themselves from threat in anxiety. You may use similar measures to protect yourself from feeling unhealthy jealousy. You reason that since you feel unhealthy jealousy about 'third person' and 'uncertainty' threats to your relationship with your partner, you'll take steps to avoid unhealthy jealousy. This involves ensuring that your partner doesn't interact with potential rivals and that you know where she (in this case) is and what she's doing.

However, this stance and the reasoning that leads you to take it are flawed and will only serve to perpetuate your tendency to feel unhealthy jealousy. This is because your unhealthy jealousy isn't based on 'third person' and 'uncertainty' threats to your relationship, but on your IBs about such threats. So if you want to deal effectively with unhealthy jealousy you need to do the following:

- Don't attempt to prevent your partner from interacting with potential rivals.
- Don't keep tabs on your partner. Allow her to do what she wants without you knowing exactly where she is, what she's doing and with whom she's interacting.
- If you actually face threats to your relationship as a result, deal with these by bringing to such situations appropriate specific versions of your general RBs so you feel healthily jealous and not unhealthily jealous about these episodes. Also, act and think in ways consistent with these specific RBs as far as possible.

Why you feel unhealthily jealous much of the time and how to deal with this

If you're particularly prone to unhealthy jealousy, you tend to make jealousy-related inferences in ambiguous situations. You do so because you hold a general IB such as: 'I must know at all times that my relationship isn't under threat. I can't bear not knowing this.'

Holding this belief, you'll assume you face a threat to your relationship in a situation of

- ambiguity – where it's not clear to you what is happening between your partner and a third person whom you see as a rival;
- uncertainty – where you don't know the whereabouts (broadly defined) of your partner.

How to deal with chronic unhealthy jealousy

To deal with chronic unhealthy jealousy, develop and apply an alternative general RB, e.g. 'I'd like to know at all times that my relationship isn't under threat, but I don't need to know this. I struggle with such uncertainty and ambiguity, but I can tolerate these unpleasant states and it's worth it to me to do so.'

Such a belief will lead you to think your relationship is under threat only where there's clear evidence for making such an inference. When there is, you need to hold a specific RB about such a threat.

How to examine the accuracy of unhealthy jealousy-related inference if necessary

If you're still unsure whether a threat exists to your relationship, answer one or more of the following questions:

- How valid is my inference that there's a threat to my relationship (for example)?
- Would an objective jury agree that there's a threat to my relationship? If not, what would their verdict be?
- Is my inference that there's a threat to my relationship realistic? If not, what is a more realistic inference?
- If I asked someone I could trust to give me an objective opinion about my inference that there's a threat to my relationship, what would that person say to me and why? What inference would he or she encourage me to make instead?
- If a friend told me he had made the same inference that he faced a threat to his relationship, what would I say to him about the validity of his inference and why? What inference would I encourage him to make instead?

Understand the thinking consequences of your IBs

When you hold a set of IBs about relationship threats and related uncertainty threats, as discussed, a consequence is that your subsequent thinking is highly distorted and skewed to the negative.

If you don't understand how your mind works in this respect, you'll get caught up in your compelling distorted thoughts, regard them as representing reality and strive to protect yourself from what you regard as real negative events rather than seeing them as highly distorted thinking consequences of IBs you've created.

However, if you do understand this phenomenon and act on this understanding, you'll trace such thinking back to the IBs that spawned it and will do one of two things (or both):

- question these IBs;
- acknowledge the existence of such distorted thinking and go about your business, neither engaging with it nor trying to eliminate it; you'll maintain this understanding no matter how compelling your distorted thoughts are.

Summary

You can make yourself less prone to unhealthy jealousy by:

- accepting yourself unconditionally for being prone to unhealthy jealousy;
- dealing effectively with your emotional problems about unhealthy jealousy;
- developing RBs enabling you to make realistic inferences at 'A' concerning threats to your relationship;
- understanding that when you hold IBs about frustration/goal

obstruction/rule transgression/disrespect or threats to your self-esteem, you'll exaggerate the nature of these inferences and its consequences. However, you will not engage with such thinking but will trace it back to the IBs that spawned it, which you'll challenge; you'll then let any remnants of such thinking be, again without engaging with it or trying to eliminate it.

In the next chapter, I deal with the deadly emotion known as unhealthy envy.

9

Dealing with unhealthy envy

This chapter outlines the RECBT view of unhealthy envy and its healthy alternative, healthy envy, showing how to deal effectively with this deadly emotion.

Understanding unhealthy envy

This section discusses the RECBT view of what happens when you make yourself unhealthily envious and how to deal effectively with this deadly emotion, using RECBT's 'ABC' model where 'A' stands for 'adversity', 'B' for beliefs and 'C' for the consequences of these beliefs. However, I will use the order 'CAB' since it's best to start with features of unhealthy envy at 'C'.

'C'

Chapter 1 explained that there are three main features of any emotional problem: feeling, behavioural and thinking. You're likely to feel unhealthily envious in several ways. Common experiences include anxiety, depression, healthy anger and rumination about what you don't have but prize. These feelings tend to interfere with your thinking clearly about what you feel unhealthily envious about and impede constructive action.

Behaviour associated with unhealthy envy

When feeling unhealthily envious, you tend to act as outlined in Table 9.1.

Thinking associated with unhealthy envy

When you feel unhealthily envious, you tend to think as outlined in Table 9.1, exaggerating what you originally felt unhealthily envious about and see as its likely consequences.

'A'

The major theme in relation to your personal domain implicated in unhealthy envy is: someone has something that you prize but don't

Table 9.1 Unhealthy envy vs healthy envy

Adversity	• Another person possesses and enjoys something desirable that you do not have.	
Belief	IRRATIONAL	RATIONAL
Emotion	Unhealthy envy	Healthy envy
Behaviour	• You verbally disparage the person who has the desired possession to others. • You verbally disparage the desired possession to others. • If you had the chance you would take away the desired possession from the other person (either so that you will have it or so that he or she is deprived of it). • If you had the chance you would spoil or destroy the desired possession so that the other person does not have it.	• You strive to obtain the desired possession if it is truly what you want.
Subsequent thinking	• You tend to denigrate in your mind the value of the desired possession and/or the person who possesses it. • You try to convince yourself that you are happy with your possessions (although you are not). • You think about how to acquire the desired possession regardless of its usefulness. • You think about how to deprive the other person of the desired possession. • You think about how to spoil or destroy the other's desired possession.	• You honestly admit to yourself that you desire the desired possession. • You are honest with yourself if you are not happy with your possessions, rather than defensively trying to convince yourself that you are happy with them when you are not. • You think about how to obtain the desired possession because you desire it for healthy reasons. • You can allow the other person to have and enjoy the desired possession without denigrating that person or the possession.

have. In unhealthy envy your focus may be on the object,[8] i.e. you think you really want the object for its own sake (object-focused unhealthy envy), or on the person who has the object, i.e. you only prize the object

---

8 I am using the word 'object' here very broadly to include anything that you prize.

because the particular person has it (person-focused unhealthy envy). The common denominator in these different types of envy is that you consider yourself to be in a state of deprivation.

As with other deadly emotions discussed in this book, perhaps with the exception of shame and guilt, these unhealthy envy-related inferences may occur in either the ego realm or the non-ego realm of your personal domain.

'B'

As Chapter 1 explained, beliefs are at the heart of the RECBT model of the emotions. Envy-related inference, on its own, doesn't explain your unhealthy envy, since, as I show, it's possible and desirable to feel healthily envious about this inference. Chapter 1 indicated that you can hold a set of IBs or RBs about adversity.

IBs about someone having something you prize but don't possess

The RECBT model of unhealthy envy is that you feel unhealthily envious about someone having something you prize but don't possess when you hold IBs about this inference. These beliefs are rigid and extreme. Please note:

- rigid beliefs are common to both ego unhealthy envy and non-ego unhealthy envy;
- self-depreciation beliefs are the main extreme beliefs in ego unhealthy envy;
- awfulizing beliefs and discomfort intolerance beliefs are the main extreme beliefs in non-ego unhealthy envy.

Understanding healthy envy

As Chapter 1 explained, when you face a negative event it's healthy for you to experience a negative emotion that helps you deal effectively with the negative event you face. This section discusses the RECBT view of healthy envy as the healthy alternative to unhealthy envy, again using the 'CABDE' order of the 'ABCDE' framework.

'C'

As explained above, there are three main features of unhealthy envy: feeling, behavioural and thinking. The same is true when you're healthily envious rather than unhealthily envious. Common experiences include concern, sadness, healthy anger and thinking about what you don't have but prize, but without rumination. Such feelings in healthy envy help you think more clearly about someone having something that you prize but don't have, and also tend to motivate you to take constructive action.

Behaviour associated with healthy envy

When healthily rather than unhealthily envious, you're motivated to strive for something you covet only if you really want it. Table 9.1 outlines the major ways you act or feel like acting when healthily envious.

Thinking associated with healthy envy

When healthily rather than unhealthily envious, you tend to think in ways designed to help you deal effectively with not having something you want that someone else has (see Table 9.1).

'A'

When healthily envious, what you feel healthily envious about is the same as what you feel unhealthily envious about, i.e. someone has something you prize but don't have. Again, your focus may be on the object, i.e. you want the object for its own sake (object-focused healthy envy), or on the person who has the object, i.e. you prize the object largely because the particular person has it (person-focused healthy envy). The common denominator in these different types of envy is again that you consider yourself to be in a state of deprivation.

'B'

When you feel healthily rather than unhealthily envious about someone having something you prize but don't possess, you do so because the beliefs you hold about these inferences are rational.

RBs about someone having something you prize but don't possess

The RECBT model of healthy envy is that you feel healthily envious about someone having something you prize but don't have when you hold RBs about these inferences. These beliefs are flexible and non-extreme. Please note:

- flexible beliefs are common to both ego healthy envy and non-ego healthy envy;
- unconditional self-acceptance beliefs are the main non-extreme beliefs in ego healthy envy;
- non-awfulizing beliefs and discomfort tolerance beliefs are also the main non-extreme beliefs in non-ego healthy envy.

How to deal with unhealthy envy

Since you make yourself unhealthily envious about someone having something you prize but don't have, your goal is to make yourself healthily envious rather than unhealthily envious about this same inference. That's why I'll be encouraging you to assume temporarily that your inference that someone has something you prize but don't have at 'A' is correct. Once you're healthily rather than unhealthily envious, you'll be in a sufficiently rational frame of mind to examine your envy-related inference. If you're unhealthily envious about this inference, you will not be objective enough while examining them. Later, I'll explain why you're prone to inferring the existence of this inference in ambiguous situations and will help you become less prone.

Ensure that you're feeling unhealthily envious and it's a problem for you

Before doing anything to try to change your feelings of unhealthy envy, ensure that you're unhealthily envious and that you see unhealthy envy is a problem for you. Otherwise, you'll resist your own efforts to help yourself.

Do you feel unhealthily envious?

People use the term 'envy' loosely; if you say you feel envious, you may or may not be experiencing the deadly version of this emotion. Determine whether you're experiencing the deadly version by consulting the behavioural and thinking consequences of both IBs and RBs about envy-related inferences. The more your behaviour and thinking match those listed in Table 9.1 as consequences of IBs, the more likely you feel/felt unhealthily envious, rather than healthily envious. Conversely, the more your behaviour and thinking match those listed as consequences of RBs, the more likely you feel/felt healthily envious rather than unhealthily envious.

Is unhealthy envy a problem for you?

Assuming you've determined that you experienced unhealthy envy rather than healthy envy, now determine whether you consider unhealthy envy is a problem you want to change. Just because your experience matches those listed in Table 9.1 as unhealthy envy doesn't mean you'll inevitably see that it's a problem for you.

If you're uncertain whether unhealthy envy is a problem for you, answer the following:

- Does my unhealthy envy help me deal effectively with someone having something I prize but don't have?

- Does my unhealthy envy help me determine whether I really want what I covet?

If you've answered 'yes' to one or both of these questions, you may be reluctant to target your unhealthy envy for change. I suggest you read the following section with an open mind, then answer two different questions.

Commit to healthy envy as a productive alternative to unhealthy envy

In any self-change venture, you need clear alternatives to problems you wish to change. Otherwise you'll be in a 'change vacuum', where you know what you don't want to feel but don't know what it would be healthy for you to feel instead. RECBT argues that when you face (or think you're facing) relationship threats and/or related uncertainty threats, the healthy alternative to feeling unhealthily envious about these inferences is to feel healthily envious about them. Table 9.1 lists the behavioural and thinking consequences of RBs about someone having something that you prize but don't have that are associated with healthy envy. If you see that these consequences help you to deal effectively with this inference, you're ready to commit yourself to feeling healthily envious rather than unhealthily envious about such an inference.

For those ambivalent about targeting unhealthy envy as a problem to change in the previous section, answer the following questions while consulting the relevant sections of Table 9.1:

- Will unhealthy envy or healthy envy help me deal more effectively with someone having something I prize but don't have?
- Which form of envy will help me think more clearly about whether I really want what I covet: unhealthy envy or healthy envy?

Hopefully, if you were ambivalent about targeting your unhealthy envy for change, you're now ready to do so and to work towards feeling healthily rather than unhealthily envious about someone having something you prize but don't have.

Identify what you're most unhealthily envious about at 'A'

If you have a problem with unhealthy envy, you're likely to experience this deadly emotion in situations where you infer that someone has something that you prize but don't have. For our purposes in this chapter, there are two realms of your personal domain:

- the ego realm, where you infer not having something you prize that someone else has as impacting on your self-esteem;

- the non-ego realm, where you infer not having something you prize that someone else has as impacting on your sense of comfort, broadly defined.

To identify what you're unhealthily envious about, ask yourself:

- What was I most unhealthily envious about in the situation I was in?
- What did the other person have that I prized but didn't possess?
- Did I envy the other person the object because of the object or the person?

Use the 'magic question' technique

If you still cannot identify your unhealthy envy-related inference, use the 'magic question' technique:

- Focus on the situation in which you felt unhealthily envious.
- Without changing the situation, ask yourself: 'What one thing would have eliminated or significantly reduced my unhealthy envy?'
- The opposite is what you were most unhealthily envious about.

Here's how Harry used this technique:

- I felt unhealthily envious when I learned my brother had a new girl-friend and had announced his engagement.
- If I had been going out with someone, I wouldn't have felt unhealth-ily envious.
- I was most unhealthily envious about my brother having a girlfriend when I don't have one.

Identify the IBs underpinning your unhealthy envy and the rational alternatives underpinning healthy envy

The RECBT model argues that not having something you prize that someone else has doesn't make you feel unhealthily envious. Rather, you make yourself unhealthily envious by holding IBs (at 'B') about this inference, and if you held RBs (also at 'B') about it instead you'd feel healthy rather than unhealthy envy.

Consequently, you should identify your IBs about your envy-related inference at 'A' and the rational alternatives to these IBs. I recommend the latter so you can derive hope that you can see that there's an alter-native to the main determining factor of your unhealthy envy.

In identifying your IBs and alternative RBs, determine whether your unhealthy envy is ego-related, impacting on your self-esteem, or non-ego-related, impacting on your sense of comfort, broadly defined, and not impacting on your self-esteem. Also determine whether your unhealthy envy is object-focused (where you're unhealthily envious because of the object rather than the person who has the object) or person-focused (where you're unhealthily envious because of the person who has the object rather than the object itself). Then do the following.

Ego unhealthy envy

If your unhealthy envy is ego-related, identify your rigid belief and self-depreciation belief about not having something you prize that someone else has at 'A'. Then identify their rational alternatives, i.e. your flexible belief and unconditional self-acceptance.

Examples of unhealthy and healthy ego envy

- Object-focused unhealthy ego envy: 'I must have the latest clothes my friends have. If I don't have them, I'm useless.'
- Object-focused healthy ego envy: 'I'd like to have the latest clothes my friends have, but I don't have to have them. If I don't have them, that is unfortunate, but it doesn't prove I'm useless. I'm an unrateable, fallible human being whether or not I have these clothes.'
- Person-focused unhealthy ego envy: 'I must have what my cousins have. If I don't, they are better than me.'
- Person-focused healthy ego envy: 'I would like to have what my cousins have, but I don't have to have it. If I don't, that would be bad, but it wouldn't prove they're better than me. I'm equal to them even though they may have more than me.'

Non-ego unhealthy envy

If your unhealthy envy is non-ego-related, identify your rigid belief and either your awfulizing belief or discomfort intolerance belief about what you were most unhealthily envious about at 'A'. Then identify their rational alternatives, i.e. your flexible belief and either your non-awfulizing belief or discomfort tolerance belief.

Examples of unhealthy and healthy non-ego envy

- Object-focused unhealthy non-ego envy: 'I must have the latest clothes my friends have. I can't stand the deprivation of not having them.'
- Object-focused healthy non-ego envy: 'I'd like to have the latest clothes my friends have, but it isn't necessary I have them. If I don't have them, it would be a struggle for me to tolerate the deprivation, but I can do so and it would be worth it to me to do so.'
- Person-focused unhealthy non-ego envy: 'I must have what my cousins have. I can't bear the inequality of not having what they have.'
- Person-focused healthy non-ego envy: 'I would like to have what my

cousins have, but I don't have to have it. It would be hard for me to put up with the resultant inequality, but I can do so and it would be in my healthy interests to do so.'

Acknowledge the 'B–C' connection

Before proceeding to question these beliefs, acknowledge the connection between your IBs (at 'B') and unhealthy envy (at 'C') and between your RBs (also at 'B') and healthy envy (at 'E') you're aiming to experience in response to your envy-related inference (at 'A').

Question your beliefs

You're now ready to question your beliefs. The purpose of the questioning process is for you to see clearly that your IBs are irrational (i.e. false, illogical and largely unhelpful) and that your alternative RBs are rational (i.e. true, logical and largely helpful).

To enable you to get the most out of the questioning process:

- Begin by questioning your rigid belief and flexible belief together. Ask yourself:
  - Which of these beliefs is true? Which is false?
  - Which of these beliefs is logical? Which is illogical?
  - Which of these beliefs is largely helpful? Which is largely unhelpful?
  Provide reasons for your answers. See Appendix 2 for suggestions concerning arguments on this issue. You'll need to tailor your arguments to the content of your beliefs.
- If your unhealthy envy is ego-based, take your self-depreciation belief and unconditional self-acceptance belief and question them by asking the same three questions as above. Again provide reasons for your answers. See Appendix 3 for suggestions concerning arguments on this issue, which have to be tailored to the content of your beliefs.
- If your unhealthy envy is non-ego-based, then either take your awfulizing belief and non-awfulizing belief or discomfort intolerance belief and discomfort tolerance belief and question the relevant pairing by asking the same three questions as above, providing reasons for your answers as before. See Appendices 4 and 5 for suggestions concerning arguments on this issue, which have to be tailored to the content of your beliefs.

Having completed this questioning process you should understand why your IBs are irrational and why the rational alternatives to these beliefs are rational, and you should be in a position to commit yourself to act and think in ways consistent with your RBs to enable you to deal effectively with whatever it was you were unhealthily envious about in the first instance.

Face your unhealthy envy-related theme in imagery

Assuming you've committed to act on your RBs (i.e. flexible belief and non-extreme belief), you must face up to someone having something you prize but don't have and learn to think rationally about it.

Until now you've worked generally in regard to your unhealthy envy-related theme, the IBs that account for your unhealthy envy and developing your alternative RBs. However, to apply your RBs in dealing with this inference, remember that since you make yourself unhealthily envious about specific events (actual or imagined), you should deal with these by rehearsing specific variants of your RBs.

The best way to do this is in specific situations in which you made yourself unhealthily envious, but you may benefit by first using imagery as follows:

- Imagine a specific situation in which you felt unhealthily envious about someone having something that you prize, but don't have, and focus, in your mind's eye, on what you felt most unhealthily envious about (i.e. your 'A').
- Focusing on 'A' while rehearsing a specific RB, try to make yourself feel healthily envious, but not unhealthily envious.
- Imagine yourself acting in ways consistent with your RB, e.g. expressing admiration for rather than denigrating the person or object concerned.
- Recognize that some of your post-belief thinking may be distorted. Respond without getting bogged down doing so. Accept the presence of any remaining distorted thoughts without engaging with them.
- Repeat the above steps until you feel sufficiently ready to put this sequence into practice in your life.

Act in ways consistent with your RBs

When you experience the emotional problem of unhealthy envy and the thoughts accompanying it, you will also experience a strong urge to act on them. If you do, you'll only serve to strengthen the IBs underpinning such behaviour. So after you have questioned your IBs and RBs as suggested above and committed yourself to strengthening your conviction in your RBs, you should act in ways that will do this and refrain from acting in ways that will do the opposite.

It's crucial to act according to the behavioural goals you identified earlier and accept that, while you do so, you'll still have the urge to act and think in unhealthy ways. Accept that this is an almost inevitable and natural part of the change process and these unhealthy urges and thoughts will eventually subside if you don't engage with them. I stress that this is difficult, but if you're clear about what you need to do and act accordingly, you'll stack the odds in favour of, rather than against, dealing effectively with your unhealthy envy.

Capitalize on what you have learned and generalize your learning

When you've acted and thought in ways consistent with your RBs, reflect on what you did and what you have learned. In particular, if you were able to face the situation where someone has something that you prize, rehearsed your specific RBs and acted in a way consistent with these beliefs, then ask yourself how you can capitalize on what you achieved and generalize your learning to similar or different unhealthy envy-related situations.

Deal with any problems facing unhealthy envy-related situations

If you experienced any problems facing a situation where someone has something that you prize, but don't possess, answer the following:

- Did I face the situation? If not, why not?
- Did I rehearse my RBs before, during or after facing the situation? If not, why not?
- Did I engage with post-belief distorted thinking? If so, why?
- Reflect on your experience and put into practice what you learned the next time you face a situation in which someone has something that you prize but lack.

Become less prone to unhealthy envy

So far I've discussed how you can help yourself deal with unhealthy envy about specified situations where someone has something that you prize but do not possess. However, what if you're particularly prone to unhealthy envy (i.e. you often focus on what others have that you lack, but think that you want, and you feel unhealthily envious about this)? I suggest the following.

Accept yourself unconditionally for being prone to unhealthy envy

If you're prone to unhealthy envy for whatever reason, you have an important choice to make at the outset: you can accept yourself unconditionally as a fallible human being, prone to experiencing unhealthy envy, or you can depreciate yourself for this proneness. Before making your choice, remember that unconditional self-acceptance doesn't mean you need to resign yourself to a lifetime of proneness to unhealthy envy. It means you're a fallible human being whether or not you're prone to unhealthy envy. It doesn't indicate that you cannot work to become less prone to this deadly emotion. Indeed, it helps you do this. If you depreciate yourself for being prone to unhealthy envy, you not only have emotional disturbance stemming from unhealthy envy proneness, you're also disturbing yourself about this disturbance: two disturbances for the price of one. So accepting yourself unconditionally for your proneness to unhealthy envy not only spares you this secondary disturbance but helps you focus on your proneness with the purpose of helping yourself become less prone.

My advice then is: choose to accept yourself unconditionally for being prone to unhealthy envy.

Deal with emotional problems about unhealthy envy

Just as you disturb yourself about being prone to unhealthy envy, you may also disturb yourself about specific instances of unhealthy envy by making yourself:

- anxious about the prospect of experiencing unhealthy envy;
- depressed about experiencing unhealthy envy;
- guilty about experiencing unhealthy envy;
- ashamed about experiencing unhealthy envy;
- unhealthily angry with yourself for making yourself unhealthily envious.

See the chapters on anxiety, depression, guilt, shame and unhealthy anger for help if you tend to disturb yourself about feeling unhealthily envious.

Develop a realistic perspective on the place of objects[9] in your life

If you want to be less prone to unhealthy envy (particularly when it's object-focused), it's important to develop a realistic perspective on the place of objects in your life. From this perspective, such objects aren't necessary to your well-being, nor can they affect your self-esteem. Once you see that such objects can only enhance your well-being if they're truly what you desire, then you'll have made yourself less vulnerable to experiencing object-focused unhealthy envy.

Make healthy comparisons

If you want to be less prone to unhealthy envy (particularly person-focused), it's important to make healthy comparisons between yourself

---

9 Please remember that I am using the term 'objects' in this chapter to refer to anything that you prize.

and others. From this perspective, you have equal worth to others and this doesn't change, even if they have something that you prize but lack. Once you see that others are advantaged when they have something that you truly value but that this doesn't affect your parity concerning your human worth, you will have made yourself less vulnerable to experiencing person-focused unhealthy envy.

Why you feel unhealthily envious much of the time and how to deal with this

If you're particularly prone to unhealthy envy, you hold a general IB such as: 'I must have what others have. If I don't, I'm less worthy and/ or I can't stand the deprivation.'

Holding this belief will lead you to focus on what others have that you don't have and think that you really want it.

How to deal with chronic unhealthy envy

To deal with this chronic sense of unhealthy envy, you need to develop and apply an alternative general RB, such as: 'I would like to have what others have, but this isn't necessary. If I don't, I'm not less worthy since my worth is fixed and doesn't vary according to my possessions. Also, I can stand the deprivation, even though it may be hard to do so.'

Such a belief will lead you to consider carefully how much you really want what others have that you don't have. It will also help you to have a balanced perspective on what you have in your life, as well as what you lack.

How to examine the strength of your desire for what others have that you prize, but don't have

When you operate according to a set of general and specific RBs with respect to what someone else has that you prize but don't have, you should be able to gauge how important the desired object truly is to you. However, if you're still unsure that you really want what others have that you prize but don't have, do the following:

- Ask yourself how strong your desire is for the prized object.
- Ask yourself whether you would still want the object if getting it didn't improve your self-esteem or make you feel better about life.
- If the other people who possess the desired object suddenly discarded it, would you still want it?
- Draw up a list of pros and cons for striving to get the object.

Understand the thinking consequences of your IBs

When you hold a set of IBs about what others have that you lack but desire, as discussed, a consequence is that your subsequent thinking is highly distorted and skewed to the negative.

If you don't understand how your mind works in this respect, then you'll get caught up in your compelling distorted thoughts, regard them as representing reality and strive to protect yourself from what you regard as real negative events, rather than seeing them as highly distorted thinking consequences of IBs you've created.

However, if you do understand this phenomenon and act on this understanding, you'll trace such thinking back to the IBs that spawned it and will do one of two things (or both):

- question these IBs;
- acknowledge the existence of such distorted thinking and go about your business while neither engaging with it nor trying to eliminate it; you'll maintain this understanding no matter how compelling your distorted thoughts are.

Summary

You can make yourself less prone to unhealthy envy by:

- accepting yourself unconditionally for being prone to unhealthy envy;
- dealing effectively with your emotional problems about unhealthy envy;
- developing a realistic perspective on the role of objects in your life;
- making comparisons between yourself and others based on the presence or absence of valued objects and not on the idea that human worth can increase or decrease depending on the ownership of these objects;
- developing RBs enabling you to think about what you have as well as what you don't have, which will enable you to be realistic about what you want in life;
- understanding that when you hold IBs about someone having what you prize but don't have, you'll exaggerate the importance of what you don't have and the consequences of not possessing it. However, you will not engage with such thinking but will trace it back to the IBs that spawned it, which you'll challenge; you'll then let any remnants of such thinking be, again without engaging with it or trying to eliminate it.

I have now reached the end of the book. I would appreciate your feedback, c/o Sheldon Press.

Appendix 1

Descriptions, foundations and illustrations
of thinking errors and their realistic and balanced alternatives

Descriptions of thinking errors and realistic and balanced alternatives

Illustrations[1]

Jumping to unwarranted conclusions

Here, when something bad happens, you make a negative interpretation and treat this as a fact even though there is no definite evidence that convincingly supports your conclusions.

'Since they have seen me fail ... [as I absolutely should not have done] ... they will view me as an incompetent worm.'

Sticking to the facts and testing out your hunches

Here, when something bad happens, you stick to the facts and resolve to test out any negative interpretations you may make which you view as hunches to be examined rather than as facts.

'Since they have seen me fail ... [as I would have preferred not to do, but do not demand that I absolutely should not have done] ... I am not sure how they will view me. I think that some will think badly of me, others will be compassionate towards me and yet others may not have noticed or be neutral about my failure. I can always ask them, if I want to know.'

All-or-none thinking

Here, you use non-overlapping black or white categories.

'If I fail at any important task ... [as I must not do] ... I will only ever fail again'

Multi-category thinking

Here, you make use of a number of relevant categories.

'If I do fail at any important task ... [as I would prefer not to do, but do not demand that I must not do] ... I may well both succeed and fail at important tasks in the future.'

Overgeneralization

Here, when something bad happens, you make a generalization from this experience that goes far beyond the data at hand.

'[My boss must like me] ... If my boss does not like me, it follows that nobody at work will like me.'

---

1 In these illustrations, the beliefs (irrational and rational) are shown in square brackets and the thinking errors and realistic and balanced alternatives are underlined.

Making a realistic generalization

Here, when something goes wrong, you make a generalization from this experience that is warranted by the data at hand.

'[I want my boss to like me, but he does not have to do so] ... If my boss does not like me, it follows that others at work may or may not like me.'

Focusing on the negative

Here, you pick out a single negative detail and dwell on it exclusively so that your vision of all reality becomes darkened, like the drop of ink that discolours the entire glass of water.

'As things are going wrong ... [as they must do and it is intolerable that they are] ... I can't see any good that is happening in my life.'

Focusing on the complexity of experiences

Here, you focus on a negative detail, but integrate this detail into the complexity of positive, negative and neutral features of life.

'As things are going wrong ... [as I prefer, but do not demand that they must not and when they do, I can bear it] ... I can see that my life is made up of the good, the bad and the neutral.'

Disqualifying the positive

Here, you reject positive experiences by insisting they "don't count" for some reason or other, thus maintaining a negative view that cannot be contradicted by your everyday experiences.

'[I absolutely should not have done the foolish things that I have done] ... When others compliment me on the good things I have done, they are only being kind to me by seeming to forget those foolish things.'

Incorporating the positive into a complex view of your experiences

Here, you accept positive experiences and locate these into the complexity of positive, negative and neutral features of life.

'[I would have preferred not to have done the foolish things that I have done, but that does not mean that I absolutely should not have done them] ... When others compliment me on the good things I have done, I can accept these compliments as being genuine even though I also did some foolish things which the others may also have recognized.'

Mind reading

Here, you arbitrarily conclude that someone is reacting negatively to you, and you don't bother to check this out. You regard your thought as a fact.

'I made some errors in the PowerPoint presentation ... [that I absolutely should not have made] ... and when I looked at my boss, I thought he was thinking how hopeless I was and therefore he did think this.'

Owning and checking one's thoughts about the reactions of others

Here, you may think someone is reacting negatively to you, but you check it out with the other person rather than regarding your thought as fact.

'I made some errors in the PowerPoint presentation ... [that I would have preferred not to have made, but that does not mean that I absolutely should not have made them] ... and when I looked at my boss I thought he was thinking that I was hopeless, but I quickly realized that this was my thought rather than his and resolved to ask him about this in the morning.'

Fortune telling

Here, you anticipate that things will turn out badly, and you feel convinced that your prediction is an already established fact.

'Because I failed at this simple task ... [which I absolutely should not have done] ... I think that I will get a very bad appraisal and thus this will happen.'

Owning and checking one's thoughts about what will happen in the future

Here, you anticipate that things may turn out badly, but you regard that as a prediction that needs examining against the available date and not as an established fact.

'Because I failed at this simple task ... [which I would have preferred not to have done, do not have to be immune from so doing] ... I may get a very bad appraisal, but this is unlikely since I have done far more good than bad at work during the last year.'

Always and never thinking

Here, when something bad happens, you conclude that it will always happen and/or the good alternative will never occur.

'Because my present conditions of living are not good ... [and they are actually intolerable because they must be better than they are] ... it follows that they'll always be this way and I'll never have any happiness.'

Balanced thinking about the past, present and future

Here, when something bad happens you recognize that while it may happen again that it is not inevitable that it will and it is very unlikely that it will always occur. Also, you recognize that the good alternative may well occur in the future and that it is very unlikely that it will never happen.

'Because my present conditions of living are not good ... [but they are tolerable because they don't have to be better than they are] ... it does not follow that they will always be that way and I can be happy again.'

Magnification

Here, when something bad happens, you exaggerate its negativity.

'I made a faux pas when introducing my new colleague ... [which I absolutely should not have done and it's awful that I did so] ... and this is will have a very negative effect on my career.'

Keeping things in realistic perspective

Here, when something bad happens, you view it in its proper perspective.

'I made a faux pas when introducing my new colleague ... [which I wish I had not made, but do not have to be exempt from making. It's bad that I did so, but hardly the end of the world] ... and while people may remember it for a day or two, I doubt that it will have much lasting impact on my career.'

Minimization

Here, you inappropriately shrink things until they appear tiny (your own desirable qualities or other people's imperfections).

'[I must do outstandingly well and I am completely useless when I do not do so] ... When I have seemingly done reasonably well, this is the result of luck and anyone could have done this. Whereas if another person had done the same thing, I would acknowledge their achievement.'

Using the same balanced perspective for self and others

Here, when you do something good and/or others do something bad, you can recognize such behaviour for what it is.

'[I want to do outstandingly well, but I do not have to do so. I am not useless when I do not do so] ... When I or someone else has seemingly done reasonably well, this may be the result of luck, but it may be because I or they fully deserved to do well.'

Emotional reasoning

Here, you assume that your negative emotions necessarily reflect the way things really are: "I feel it, therefore it must be true."

'Because I have performed so poorly ... [as I absolutely should not have done] ... I feel like everybody will remember my poor performance and my strong feeling proves that they will.'

Sound reasoning based on thinking and feeling

Here when you experience emotions, your reason is sound about what these emotions and the accompanying thinking might mean.

'Because I have performed so poorly ... [as I wish, but do not demand that I absolutely should not have done] ... I think and feel that people will have different responses to my performance: some negative and nasty, some compassionate and empathic and some neutral and this is probably the case.'

Personalization

Here, when a negative event occurs involving you which you may or may not be primarily responsible for, you see yourself definitely as the cause of it.

'I am involved in a group presentation and things are not going well ... [Since I am acting worse than I absolutely should act] ... and the audience is laughing, I am sure they are laughing only at me.'

Making a realistic attribution

Here, when a negative event occurs involving you which you may or may not be primarily responsible for, you acknowledge that you may be the cause of it, but you don't assume that you definitely are. Rather, you view the event from the whole perspective before making an attribution of cause which is likely to be realistic.

'I am involved in a group presentation and things are not going well ... [Since I am acting worse than I would like to do, but do not demand that I must do] ... and the audience is laughing, I am not sure who or what they are laughing at and indeed, some might be laughing with us and not at us.'

Appendix 2

Reasons why rigid beliefs are false, illogical and have largely unhealthy consequences and flexible beliefs are true, logical and have largely healthy consequences

Rigid belief

A rigid belief is false

For such a demand to be true the demanded conditions would already have to exist when they do not. Or as soon as you make a demand then these demanded conditions would have to come into existence. Both positions are clearly false or inconsistent with reality.

A rigid belief is illogical

A rigid belief is based on the same desire as a flexible belief but is transformed as follows:

'I prefer that x happens (or does not happen) . . . and therefore this absolutely must (or must not) happen.'

The first ['I prefer that x happens (or does not happen . . .)'] is not rigid, but the second ['. . . and therefore this must (or must not) happen'] is rigid. As such a rigid belief is illogical since one cannot logically derive something rigid from something that is not rigid.

A rigid belief has largely unhealthy consequences

A rigid belief has largely unhealthy consequences because it tends to lead to unhealthy negative emotions, unconstructive behaviour and highly distorted and biased subsequent thinking when the person is facing an adversity.

Flexible belief

A flexible belief is true

A flexible belief is true because its two component parts are true. You can prove that you have a particular desire and can provide reasons why you want what you want. You can also prove that you do not have to get what you desire.

A flexible belief is logical

A flexible belief is logical since both parts are not rigid and thus the second component logically follows from the first. Thus, consider the following flexible belief:

'I prefer that x happens (or does not happen) . . . but this does not mean that it must (or must not) happen.'

The first component ['I prefer that x happens (or does not happen . . .)'] is not rigid and the second ['. . . but this does not mean that it must (or must not happen)'] is also non-rigid. Thus, a flexible belief is logical because it comprises two non-rigid parts connected together logically.

A flexible belief has largely healthy consequences

A flexible belief has largely healthy consequences because it tends to lead to healthy negative emotions, constructive behaviour and realistic and balanced subsequent thinking when the person is facing an adversity.

Appendix 3

Reasons why depreciation beliefs are false, illogical and have largely unhealthy consequences and acceptance beliefs are true, logical and have largely healthy consequences

Depreciation belief

A depreciation belief is false

When you hold a depreciation belief in the face of your adversity, this belief is based on the following ideas which are false:

- A person (self or other) or life can legitimately be given a single global rating that defines their or its essence and the worth of a person or of life is dependent upon conditions that change (e.g. my worth goes up when I do well and goes down when I don't do well).
- A person or life can be rated on the basis of one of his or her or its aspects.

Both of these ideas are patently false and thus your depreciation belief is false.

A depreciation belief is illogical

A depreciation belief is based on the idea that the whole of a person or of life can logically be defined by one of their or its parts. Thus:

x is bad . . . and therefore I am bad.

This is known as the part-whole error which is illogical.

A depreciation belief has largely unhealthy consequences

A depreciation belief has largely unhealthy consequences because it tends to lead to unhealthy negative emotions, unconstructive behaviour and highly distorted and biased subsequent thinking when the person is facing an adversity.

Acceptance belief

An acceptance belief is true

When you hold an acceptance belief in the face of your adversity, this belief is based on the following ideas which are true:

- A person (self or other) or life cannot legitimately be given a single global rating that defines their or its essence and their or its worth, as far as they or it have it, is not dependent upon conditions that change (e.g. my worth stays the same whether or not I do well).
- Discrete aspects of a person, and life can be legitimately rated, but a person or life cannot be legitimately rated on the basis of these discrete aspects.

Both of these ideas are patently true and thus your acceptance belief is true.

An acceptance belief is logical

An acceptance belief is based on the idea that the whole of a person or of life cannot be defined by one or more of their or its parts. Thus:

x is bad, but this does not mean that I am bad, I am a fallible human being even though x occurred.

Here the part-whole illogical error is avoided. Rather it is held that the whole incorporates the part which is logical.

An acceptance belief has largely healthy consequences

An acceptance belief has largely healthy consequences because it tends to lead to healthy negative emotions, constructive behaviour and realistic and balanced subsequent thinking when the person is facing an adversity.

Appendix 4

Reasons why awfulizing beliefs are false, illogical and have largely unhealthy consequences and non-awfulizing beliefs are true, logical and have largely healthy consequences

Awfulizing belief

An awfulizing belief is false

When you hold an awfulizing belief about your adversity, this belief is based on the following ideas:

- Nothing could be worse;
- The event in question is worse than 100% bad; and
- No good could possibly come from this bad event.

All three ideas are patently false and thus your awfulizing belief is false.

An awfulizing belief is illogical

An awfulizing belief is based on the same evaluation of badness as a non-awfulizing belief, but is transformed as follows:

'It is bad if x happens (or does not happen) . . . and therefore it is awful if it does happen (or does not happen).'

The first component ['It is bad if x happens (or does not happen . . .)'] is non-extreme, but the second ['. . . and therefore it is awful if it does (or does not) happen'] is extreme. As such, an awfulizing belief is illogical since one cannot logically derive something extreme from something that is non-extreme.

An awfulizing belief has largely unhealthy consequences

An awfulizing belief has largely unhealthy consequences because it tends to lead to unhealthy negative emotions, unconstructive behaviour and highly distorted and biased subsequent thinking when the person is facing an adversity.

Non-awfulizing belief

A non-awfulizing belief is true

When you hold a non-awfulizing belief about your adversity, this belief is based on the following ideas:

- Things could always be worse;
- The event in question is less than 100% bad; and
- Good could come from this bad event.

All three ideas are clearly true and thus your non-awfulizing belief is true.

A non-awfulizing belief is logical

A non-awfulizing belief is logical since both parts are non-rigid and the second component logically follows from the first. Thus, consider following non-awfulizing belief:

'It is bad if x happens (or does not happen) . . . but it is not awful if x happens (or does not happen).'

The first component ['It is bad if x happens (or does not happen . . .)'] is non-extreme and the second ['. . . but it is not awful if it does (or does not) happen'] is also non-extreme. Thus, a non-awfulizing belief is logical because it comprises two non-extreme parts connected together logically.

A non-awfulizing belief has largely healthy consequences

A non-awfulizing belief has largely healthy consequences because it tends to lead to healthy negative emotions, constructive behaviour and realistic and balanced subsequent thinking when the person is facing an adversity.

Appendix 5

Discomfort intolerance beliefs and
discomfort tolerance beliefs

Discomfort intolerance belief

A discomfort intolerance belief is false

When you hold a discomfort intolerance belief about your adversity, this belief is based on the following ideas which are all false:

- I will die or disintegrate if the discomfort continues to exist;
- I will lose the capacity to experience happiness if the discomfort continues to exist;
- Even if I could tolerate it, the discomfort is not worth tolerating.

All three ideas are patently false and thus your discomfort intolerance belief is false.

A discomfort intolerance belief is illogical

A discomfort intolerance belief is based on the same sense of struggle as a discomfort tolerance belief, but is transformed as follows:

'It would be difficult for me to tolerate it if x happens (or does not happen) . . . and therefore it would be intolerable.'

The first component ['It would be difficult for me to tolerate it if x happens (or does not happen . . .)'] is non-extreme, but the second ['. . . and therefore it would be intolerable'] is extreme. As such, a discomfort intolerance belief is illogical since one cannot logically derive something extreme from something that is non-extreme.

Discomfort tolerance belief

A discomfort tolerance belief is true

When you hold a discomfort tolerance belief about your adversity, this belief is based on the following ideas which are all true:

- I will struggle if the discomfort continues to exist, but I will neither die nor disintegrate;
- I will not lose the capacity to experience happiness if the discomfort continues to exist, although this capacity will be temporarily diminished; and
- The discomfort is worth tolerating.

All three ideas are patently true and thus your discomfort tolerance belief is true.

A discomfort tolerance belief is logical

A discomfort tolerance belief is logical since both parts are non-extreme and thus the second component logically follows from the first. Thus, consider following discomfort tolerance belief:

'It would be difficult for me to tolerate it if x happens (or does not happen) . . . but it would not be intolerable (and it would be worth tolerating).'

The first component ['It would be difficult for me to tolerate it if x happens (or does not happen . . .)'] is non-extreme and the second ['. . . but it would not be intolerable (and it would be worth tolerating)'] is also non-extreme. Thus, a discomfort tolerance belief is logical because it comprises two non-extreme parts connected together logically.

A discomfort intolerance belief has largely unhealthy consequences

A discomfort intolerance belief has largely unhealthy consequences because it tends to lead to unhealthy negative emotions, unconstructive behaviour and highly distorted and biased subsequent thinking when the person is facing an adversity.

A discomfort tolerance belief has largely healthy consequences

A discomfort tolerance belief has largely healthy consequences because it tends to lead to healthy negative emotions, constructive behaviour and realistic and balanced subsequent thinking when the person is facing an adversity.

Index